YOUR LIBRARY MILLAGE AT WORK
PORT HUI
ST. CLAIR C(

MW00909131

UNDERSTANDING MENTAL ILLNESS
Comprehensive & Jargon Free

6th EDITION

MARIANNE RICHARDS

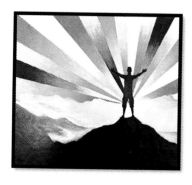

**THIS BOOK WAS
DONATED BY:**

**St. Clair County
Community
Mental Health**

Gift of Knowledge 2016

JUN   2016

www.inspirationWorks4U.co.uk

© Copyright Marianne Richards 2015

6th edition

First Published 2000 Straightforward, Brighton.
Reprinted 2002, 2004, 2006. 2012

Illustrations by Mole Graphics and the author.

The right of Marianne Richards to be identified as author of this work
has been asserted by her in accordance with Copyright, Designs and
Patents Act 1988

ISBN-13: 978-1517443474
ISBN-10: 1517443474

All rights reserved. No reproduction, copy or transmission of this
publication may be made without written permission. No paragraph
of this publication may be reproduced, copied or transmitted save
with the written permission or in accordance with the provisions of
the Copyright Act 1956 (as amended). Any person who does any
unauthorized act in relation to this publication may be liable to
criminal prosecution and civil claims for damage.

Whilst every care has been taken to ensure the accuracy of this work,
the author or publisher cannot accept responsibility for loss
occasioned by any person acting or refraining to act as a result of any
statement contained within this book.

Dedication

David Richards
Hoping you found your way too.

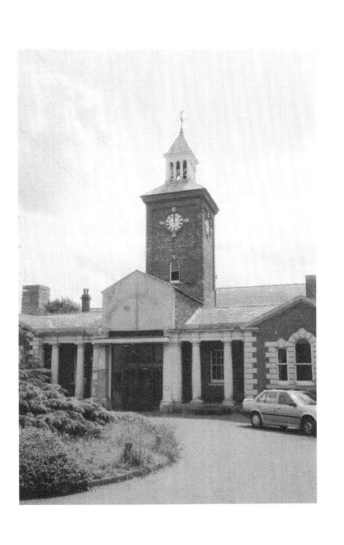

Marianne Richards holds a Masters Degree in Mental Health Practice, Diploma in Ericksonian Solution-Focused Therapy and Certificate in Behavioural Family Therapy, as well as a media qualification. She worked in private practice and the NHS as a Counsellor and Mental Health Worker for two decades, gaining many testimonials from patients and Doctors. In 2000 she was offered her first publishing contract and received professional acclaim for her layman guides to adult mental illness.

After being bullied out of her NHS career, Marianne was diagnosed with clinical depression and had a breakdown. During this time, she was diagnosed with high functioning autism (Asperger Syndrome), the stress having triggered the florid symptoms which enabled diagnosis. These experiences now inform her writing.

Throughout these ordeals, Marianne found much solace in a life-long love of writing. She began to study other forms of writing, supporting herself in a variety of jobs from security guard to saleswoman. In 2014, Marianne set up micro-publishing house, InspirationWorks4U, with the aim of writing / publishing inspiring, entertaining works in the genres of historical fiction, drama and poetry. Her interests outside writing and research include, gardening, DIY, computers - and 'anything new'.

Praise for Marianne's mental health books:

'The author gives an intelligent overview of mental health problems and a valuable perspective on [mental health] services. Highly recommended for lay readers, carers, patients and newly qualified professionals.' –
Dr Ernest Gralton, Fellow, Royal College of Psychiatrists
                *

'This is the type of thing you don't read about in the standard texts.'
Dr Kate Kerr, Senior House Officer in Psychiatry
                *

'Written in simple terms to make it .. understandable by the lay reader. Of great help to those [with] mental ill health or their carers.'
Dr Peter Ager, Senior Partner [retired]
                *

"This highly readable book…is a valuable contribution to the understanding and acceptance of mental illness. I recommend this book to anyone who has an interest [in] mental illness.. Counsellors.. and trainees.'
Marie Anderson, BACP Accredited Counsellor & Tutor

UNDERSTANDING MENTAL ILLNESS

CONTENTS

		pp
Introduction		xiii
Ch1. Drawing the Line: What is 'Sanity'?		1
Ch 2. Mental Health & Communities		13
Ch 3. Mental Illness to 17th century		23
Ch 4. Mental Illness 18th to 20th Century		33
Ch 5. The Mental Health Act 1983		49
Ch 6. From Detection to Diagnosis		55
Ch 7. Non Medical Therapists - Talking Cures		59
Ch 8. Medical Practitioners		65
Ch. 9 Modern Medical Treatments		69
Ch 10. Pen Portraits of Therapists		87
Ch 11. Institutional Care & Support Groups		105
Ch 12. Case Histories		111
Ch 13. Social & Complementary Approaches		143
Ch 14. Stress		155
Further Information		171
Glossary		177
Index		183

ILLUSTRATIONS

pp

Continuum of Mental Illness	5
Insane or Sane	11
Balanced Personality	15
Social problems of Mental Illness	17
Culture and Diagnosis	19
Water Tower of Victorian Asylum	21
Scapegoat System	26
Mandela	29
Montage: St John's Asylum	35
Conscious and Unconscious Mind	41
Medical, Talking Cures & Alternative Therapies	63
Mental Health Staff	67
Brain Chemistry Imbalance	71
The Human Brain 1	73
The Human Brain 2	75
Process of a Drug Trial, 1	78
Process of a Drug Trial, 2	79
Process of a Drug Trial, 3	80
Drug Categories	83
Therapeutic Communities	109
Brief Psychotic Disorder	113
Prometheus – After Depression	117
Mood Cycles	127
Phobia	135
Psychological Balance	147
Keys to Mental Health	153
Fight, Flight, Freeze	157
Modern Stress	159
Personal Resources	169

Introduction

By agreement with Emerald/Straightforward, I am publishing this 6th edition in my new micro-publishing house, InspirationWorks4U.

This book is a wide ranging primer. My intended readers are newly-diagnosed patients, carers, volunteers, new professionals who need a brief outline (medics, forces, police) as well as avid searchers of new knowledge. It is not intended as self-diagnosis or self-treatment. I encourage anyone worried about symptoms to see their GP. I have written in a jargon-free style with a comprehensive glossary. There is a reading list with websites and support organisations.

The book begins with a brief overview of the history of mental illness and how its detection, diagnosis and treatment depend upon the prevailing beliefs of society. I explain why people with mental illness have been variously feared, revered or ignored throughout history. Although some symptoms might appear bizarre or frightening, I show how these link and mirror normal (neuro typical) behaviours.

Mental illness is surprisingly common. Indeed, anyone might undergo an episode given certain circumstances, which tends to surprise readers. This is not a cause for panic but shows how the perception of mental illness (a very wide field) has been distorted by narrow and sensationalist press coverage. The events most commonly reported are suicide and murder, which has led to excessive fear about depression and schizophrenia. The latter is often confused with the relatively rare psychopathic personality disorder. Most symptoms are controlled by effective modern drug treatments. I will explain how new drugs are trialled and how they work.

Although stress is not a major mental illness, it is common among patients as well as carers. For this reason, this subject has a place in my book. I also include an overview of complementary treatments. Many of these are untested but some have anecdotal evidence of effectiveness. There is some research in this area, as I explain later but complementary treatments are unsuitable for psychotic symptoms, except as stress relief. All case histories are fictional. Every experience of mental illness and response to treatment is individual, which makes diagnosis very difficult (as I will explain).

I hope you enjoy reading my book.

Marianne Richards, MSc. DipTHP
September 2015

Chapter 1
Drawing the Line - What is 'Sanity'?

Content:
Intolerance and Prejudice
Moral Panics
Exclusion and Mental Illness
Language or Labelling
Feared Mental Illnesses
Exercise
Parameters for Acceptable Behaviour
Definition of States Requiring Intervention
Drawing the line - Sanity and Insanity

Mental illness is hard to understand, even if you have experienced it. In making the attempt, it is important to ignore the unfortunate backcloth of pre-conceived ideas by ignorant others. It is also vital to understand the difficulties of diagnosis, from the professional point of view. This chapter addresses both issues.

Intolerance and Prejudice

Throughout history, individuals who have not conformed to the expectations of society (or their tribe) risked exclusion. Wearing unconventional clothing, using language or behaviour different to that commonly used in the group, or rejecting accepted politics has always put the perpetrator at risk of ridicule, stigmatization or even death, depending on the tolerance levels of their society.

In the sixteenth century, from Britain to America, millions of innocent men and women were charged with witchcraft, risking torture, imprisonment and terrible punishments if found guilty. The Catholic Church at that time wielded huge power and witch hunting was a way of maintaining it, through intimidation and fear. Town and country folk were made terrified of devils and hell by preachers and easily subdued. The infamous Catholic Inquisitions wielded terrifying power in these primitive, illiterate communities, steeped in a common fear of being afflicted with illness or having crops ruined by witches and devils. Equally, an accusation of witchcraft could be brought through spite. Anyone who offended a neighbour risked being falsely

1

accused. These unfortunates stood little chance of survival against the dreadful tortures or the absurd 'test' of ducking in a pond (where to float mean guilt and to sink meant innocence but certain death). If relatives offered comfort to their relatives at the stake, they too risked implication. It was a time when women feared growing old lest their senile looks or skin tags marked them out for accusations.

Try this quiz to see if you are the sort of person who might have been accused of witchcraft: [note – site was available at time of download on 8/9/2015]

http://www.historyextra.com/witchtest

For witchcraft, substitute the terms scapegoating, bullying or marginalising, which are the modern equivalents. Perhaps not unsurprisingly, given I have experienced being bullied, I came out as a 'yes' in the test! Solitary females, particularly if successful or in any way unusual, are vulnerable to this kind of nastiness.

Sad to say, among certain communities which remain medieval in outlook and discourage education – that is, those who wish to retain personal power not reduce suffering among their community – the fear of witchcraft remains. Shockingly, this is not only in third world despotic states, but extends among immigrants who chose to cling to old beliefs. You may remember horrific cases of children murdered by relatives, who claimed witchcraft had been detected. Or, of course, there are the abhorrent murders committed by thug jihadists, who, like Inquisitions, claim to work on the side of God.

Non-conforming individuals risk exclusion for much the same reasons as their sixteenth century forbears - fear, envy, spite, scapegoating and ignorance. With the current fear of terrorism, certain groups are still stigmatized, rather than perceiving that it is a small number of power-mad individuals causing havoc in the name of an adopted cause. When things go wrong, it is easier to blame an individual or marginalised group, rather than deal with the underlying issues. This is why this sort of behaviour continues.

Group behaviour was first analyzed by Sigmund Freud, Carl Jung and their descendants, who uncovered many of the often unconscious reasons why humans can be cruel and irrational. The purpose of rejecting what is claimed to be 'abnormal behaviour', 'strange appearance' or 'odd opinions' serves to confirm the identity and safety of a group, thus allowing them to justify cruelty. On the other hand, awareness that something unusual is happening functions as a warning of impending attack – just as screeching among gorillas signals the rest of the tribe to scatter.

Recognition of non conforming behaviour serves a useful purpose; acting upon it irrationally does not. Whilst unwarranted exclusion exists in myriad forms, those with emotional intelligence know why they do what they do, and it is usually to do with greed and power.

Moral Panics

Though cheap travel has helped to spread international culture, group pressure often precludes individual effort to reduce fear. Any irrational fear displayed by a group is referred to as a *moral panic*. A good example is Isis, with its culture-destroying, self-serving moral righteousness against all who fail to support its archaic systems. Genuine Moslems insist these people have nothing to do with Islam but only hi-jack its name. Moral panics are at odds with genuine religion, all of which preach tolerance and humanity.

Murder often triggers moral panics, particularly when linked to mental illness. In the press, a murder committed by someone with schizophrenia formerly triggered headlines like 'madman' or 'maniac' or 'psycho', usually attached to a cynical campaign to make that newspaper look good i.e. 'make our streets safer' and implying that such people had best be 'locked away'. Thanks to work by the Royal College of Psychiatrists, the days of such headlines are largely history. However moral panics still thrive when societies feel threatened by attack or when resources are limited.

Societies are often caught unawares by their own panics. In the UK a retired school master was wrongly accused of murdering a young female. The man in question sported bushy white hair and was what might be construed as eccentric (= different to the 'norm'). Accusers indulged in public tittle-tattle about his mannerisms, habits and social behaviour, based on irrational fears. Such was the moral panic, the man went into hiding. When the real murderer was caught, he reappeared. His long hair cut, he wore a suit and walked next to a grim-faced barrister. Same man, but viewed very differently by accusers who by then had disappeared into the woodwork. The BBC docu-drama, *The Lost Honour of Christopher Jefferies*, makes interesting, if sobering, viewing.

On the other hand, a mass murderer nearly got away with his crimes because he appeared the model of a caring Physician. Dr Harold Shipman, respected GP of long standing, worked for decades

3

alongside doctors, nurses and pathologists. For years the elderly were entrusted to his care by unwitting relatives. Shipman, a pillar of society, made public interviews about the treatment of the mentally ill. One day it struck an observant undertaker there had been an extraordinary number of funerals among Shipman's patients. Although charged for a small number of murders, a subsequent public enquiry suggested the number ranged between 250 and 400, making Shipman the country's most prolific serial-killer.

Shipman was eventually diagnosed with several serious personality disorders, but not insanity. Those with personality disorders are not aware they have the condition. It remains a moral issue, how far is someone guilty of crime when they do not perceive it as such.

It is perhaps a sobering fact that most murders are committed by sane people, not those diagnosed with mental illness. And psychopathic personality disorder is relatively rare.

Exclusion and Mental Illness

Up to the early 20th century, individuals with mental disorders were incarcerated in Asylums, usually sited on the edge of villages. These were not only people with active mental illness but so-called *social misfits* whose only problem was eccentricity or minor social aberrations. I met a man who had been committed by his parents because he stole a bicycle and it was common to commit single women who became pregnant. These unfortunates spent all their lives in institutions. So did the Queen's cousins, Nerissa and Katherine Bowes-Lyon, who were both born severely mentally disabled. Though officially listed in Burkes's peerage as having died, they lived all their lives in institutions, not receiving presents or visits according to staff. Such was the prevailing attitude, though their aunt, the Queen Mother, was patron of Mencap at that time. A BBC documentary, The Queen's Hidden Cousins, was made about them in 2011, provoking much anger and denial on both sides.

In the 1970's the UK Care in the Community Act forced Asylums to close. Patients were sent to live in social housing. Whilst there were instances of acceptance and tolerance, others became hostile. In the days of the asylums, those who lived and worked in local communities were understanding of their asylum-patient neighbours, because they grew familiar with florid symptoms. Though patients wanderered the village, they returned to the Asylum at night and were locked in.

Continuum of mental illness

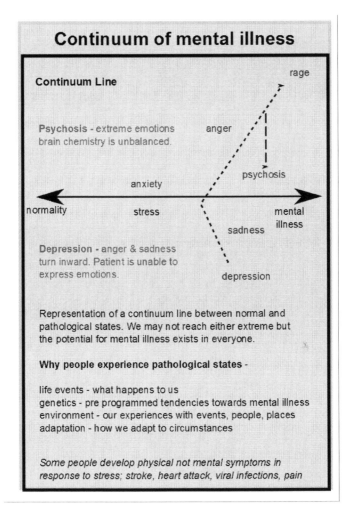

Continuum Line

rage

Psychosis - extreme emotions
brain chemistry is unbalanced.

anger

psychosis

anxiety

normality   stress   mental
                                                        illness

sadness

Depression - anger & sadness
turn inward. Patient is unable to
express emotions.

depression

Representation of a continuum line between normal and
pathological states. We may not reach either extreme but
the potential for mental illness exists in everyone.

Why people experience pathological states -

life events - what happens to us
genetics - pre programmed tendencies towards mental illness
environment - our experiences with events, people, places
adaptation - how we adapt to circumstances

Some people develop physical not mental symptoms in
response to stress; stroke, heart attack, viral infections, pain

5

With the closure of asylums, ex patients were sent into the community with little support, spending most of the day alone. A major flaw in the Care in the Community Act was lack public education about enduring mental illness. With no such knowledge, the community were left with understandable fear and prejudice. It is easy to criticise. Having lived close by neighbours with mental health problems, mostly undiagnosed, I understand some of the day to day irritations and frustrations. A return to the 'bin' system is impossible but perhaps the answer is half-way, something like a therapeutic community [see later chapter]. A very tiny number of patients represent danger if not constantly medicated and overseen. But if your family is harmed, this statistic is less meaningful. There is no complete answer but knowledge is comforting; like knowing there are very few plane crashes.

Language or Labelling

When a group of people are bent on excluding another, the first trait that is accentuated is the difference between the group and 'it'. One of the first phenomena is the use of negative words or language to describe the individual (or group). Then come false accusations (blaming or scapegoating). For example, Jews in Nazi run Germany were accused of creating the poor social conditions in the German nation, a fear successfully exploited by Hitler and his thugs.

A language develops which stigmatizes the individual. For example the derogatory term 'schizo' rather than 'a person diagnosed with schizophrenia'. Using the word 'schizo' implies this person has no identity outside their label. There may be periods when the illness is dormant so it is folly, as well as unkind, to define a person by their illness. Certainly I have been stigmatised by my autism, among people ignorant of what it means or even how I experience it (as in mental illness, veryone with autism has different experiences and different ways of expressing or coping).

The diagnosis of schizophrenia was at one time tantamount to social suicide. Labelling is helpful only for psychiatric diagnosis. Giving a name to a disorder allows preventative action to be taken – it is not meant to define a person's life.

Labelling extends to cases those commit suicide, whether or not they had active mental illness. As well as the erroneous view that people who commit suicide are selfish, they have been cruelly mocked on social websites. To counter this, there is a growing understanding of the mind state known as depression. Depression is a serious mental illness, which untreated can lead to suicide. Feeling suicidal is a phenomenon of a medical illness, not a choice. It is treatable, can be difficult to treat, and sadly can lead to loss of life. This is explored in a later chapter.

The 21ˢᵗ century view veers away from diagnostic labels and toward identifying and treating symptoms. Thus, someone might experience hallucinations and delusions (psychosis or breakdown), receive treatment then return to life untainted by a psychiatric label. Many women have breakdowns after childbirth, but no one would label all mothers psychotic, would they?

No one remains neuro-typical their whole life. We fluctuate along a median line from mental health to mental ill health. It is in everyone's interest to prevent unfair and damaging labelling, still less hostile prejudice. The human mind is a marvellous machine, but finely tuned. Imagine all those lovely neurons, firing electrical currents and making new connections. Small wonder that occasionally a link breaks down.

Feared Mental Illnesses

A tiny number of people with mental illness are dangerous because the nature of their illness makes it likely they will commit criminal acts. But, there are very few murderous psychopaths. A psychopath is born without moral capacity and cannot be 'blamed' for actions in a moral sense. Nevertheless murderous psychopaths must be locked up for the safety of the community. There is as yet no cure for this condition but there is a treatment regime for managing this disorder. Even at Broadmoor or Carstairs there is hope. And remember, these are not only prison-asylums, but people's lifelong homes. These are humans too, though this fact is often brushed under the carpet.

A small number of people with schizophrenia might fail to take medication, often because they believe there is nothing wrong with them. They can commit dangerous acts under the influence of powerful delusions. However, the vast majority with schizophrenia live successfully in the community, thanks to medication. I would rather live next door to someone with controlled schizophrenia than the anti social neighbour from hell, wouldn't you?

John Nash the great mathematician (his story is told in the film *A Beautiful Mind*) developed schizophrenia during his teens. John went on to life a full life with a happy marriage. He was recognized for his academic work by being awarded the Nobel Memorial Prize in Economic Sciences. In the days before medication, John Nash overcame his symptoms by using his powerful logic to distinguish reality from hallucinations. However this self treatment was unique. Modern medication brought great relief to those suffering the disabling psychoses connected with schizophrenia.

In conclusion, contrary to popular belief, few people with enduring mental illness are dangerous. There are far more 'bad' than 'mad' people in the world. Even among neuro-typicals there are eruptions of greed, revenge, envy, spite and murderous rage. Lately, a spate of family men under financial duress murdered their wives and children before committing suicide. None of these men were diagnosed with a major mental illness; it was an extreme form of stress.

Knowledge breeds tolerance. Few people realize how common mental illness is; that there are many types with varying severity; that episodes of illness flourish and disappear; still less that a large percentage of those diagnosed with major mental illnesses live normal lives. That is the success of medication, treatment and, still more, the enlightened view of (most) societies.

Exercise
Part 1
In a busy street you see a man dressed in white robes muttering and pointing at the sky. A crowd gathers. Some people laugh, others turn away and continue shopping. A group of tourists take photographs. The Police arrive and arrest him. Because he resists they handcuff him. This makes him angry; he shouts and foams at the mouth.

Several witnesses attend a Court hearing where the man is charged with creating a public nuisance and resisting arrest. Consider what you have read and answer the following:

Would you consider this man's behaviour rational?

- Have you any sympathy?
- Would you try to help or turn away?

Part 2
Consider the above questions, under the following conditions - this person was:
- under the influence of drugs
- a classical musician who has had too much to drink

- a young man drunk on his coming of age
- seriously mentally incapacitated
- physically disabled through a car accident
- epileptic
- speaking in a religious fervour
- in a brief psychotic episode (nervous breakdown)

Which conditions would make you feel sympathetic, less likely to want the man locked up? Which do not change your opinion? Do you believe him insane?

Part 3

Our first witness says the man is dangerous and should be imprisoned. He maliciously claims the man hit someone. Another witness says this is not true; the man was reacting to someone lunging at him. The third witness is a Psychiatrist who suspects the man has schizophrenia and recommends he is detained in a secure Hospital for observation. The fourth witness is the leader of an Arts Group who has seen the man performing in a troupe of Street Actors.

Our final witness is late. He rushes in with three other devotees. He translates for the Court that the man is their friend. They are a sect visiting a relative. In the cell their friend suffered a fit. The men are angry their friend has been maltreated. The man could not speak English and no translator was available.

It is easy to make judgements and read people through the lens of personal prejudice. Those with mental symptoms are more likely to be attacked or shunned because their symptoms are not understood and therefore feared. The basis of understanding is knowledge and at last this is being taken seriously.

Parameters for Acceptable Behaviour
Place

The robed man's behaviour took place in public. His actions were not compatible with what was acceptable in a public place. What is acceptable at an arts festival, opera house, formal dinner and a private home varies. Certain behaviours are acceptable depending upon where they are committed and for what reason.

Time

If the man continued to display this behaviour for hours or days would it increase the likelihood of his being diagnosed insane? If this behaviour stopped and he walked away, would the problem remain? Perhaps a time frame is also relevant.

Effect on Others

Our friend provoked many reactions. Whilst some experienced him as a benign he appears to have upset others. Perhaps the effect on other people is important to consider.

Ability to Survive

How long is it before a stray person is deemed incapable and taken into care? If this had been a child the time frame would be shorter. The ability of the person to survive seems to be a factor.

Definition of States Requiring Intervention

Using the above examples, a person with mental illness warranting treatment in hospital can be defined as someone who:

- acts in a manner not befitting the place
- demonstrates disturbing behaviour over time
- creates a justified adverse reaction in others
- appears incapable of looking after him/her self

In fact these are the parameters defined by the Mental Health Act 1983. Though now defunct, it is important to understand what it meant in the context of major mental illness.

Look at the diagram on the next page where I describe several people perceiving the same image. Although the answers are not definitive, I hope this offers an insight into the importance of taking culture, belief, personal life circumstances and character into consideration, when professionals make a diagnosis.

Drawing the line - Sanity and Insanity

In this context, I use the term insanity to describe a pathological state. Some Psychiatrists, notably R D Laing, questioned whether mental illness is a social construct. That is, does 'insanity' exist if there is no one to observe it? Consider this metaphor.

- If a man living alone on an island became psychotic, could his extraordinary perceptions be described as sane?
- If someone with different perceptions joins him, who is regarded as sane and who deluded - or are both realities sane / insane?
- How many people have to live on this island, before one reality is accepted and thereby defines sanity?

Insane or Sane?

PSYCHOTIC		SPIRITUAL
CREATIVE	?	NORMAL
IMAGINATIVE		ECCENTRIC

Using the adjectives above; apply one to each person described below. Reconsider your response after reading the contextual explanations at the bottom of this diagram.

1. Andrew: "Virgin Mary was watching TV in my room."
2. Maureen: "Virgin Mary said 'happy birthday!' to me."
3. John:"Virgin Mary disguises herself as a nun."
4. Stella: "I saw someone dressed like Virgin Mary."
5. Giovanni: "I paint my vision of Virgin Mary."
6. Bernie: "Virgin Mary appeared to me in a cave."

CONTEXTTUAL EXPLANATIONS

Andrew : PSYCHOTIC - Andrew is hallucinating
Maureen : IMAGINATIVE - Maureen is a child
John : ECCENTRIC - John is an eccentric thinker
Stella : NORMAL - Stella has seen an actress
Giovanni : CREATIVE - Giovanni paints icons
Bernie : SPIRITUAL - Bernadette is a Catholic saint

It is possible to define insanity as 'extraordinary perceptions which other people do not share'. Extraordinary perception is a less prejudicial expression for insanity or madness. If all extraordinary behaviour was classed as insanity, then the religious experiences of hermits and saints would be interpreted as symptoms of madness and not divine inspiration. If you suggested to a spiritual person their vision was only a hallucination and should be medicated with Haloperidol, you would certainly offend.

If a scientist believes eternal life possible and has a plan to advance this reality, he may be thought eccentric but this does not make him insane. The scientist I refer to is Dr Aubrey de Grey, an intelligent computer expert who has been offered a large grant to research his fancy, so someone takes him seriously. Perhaps insanity is also to do with levels of tolerance and knowledge.

In conclusion

Our culture has a strong influence in defining the reality we live in. Much of what might appear strange is not always the problem of the individual, but the perception of vociferous others. Stigmatisation, labelling, blaming are the result of moral panics without cause. However, labelling is also a positive trait which draws together a community in the face of war; for example, Churchill's propaganda.

Although it is known mental illness can be worsened by the stress of living in a community, positive reactions from a community can also be the root of healing. Understanding, harmony and tolerance help stabilize and reduce symptoms.

Chapter 2
Mental Illness & Communities

Content:
Education
East and West
Evidence Based Treatments
Stress of Living in Communities
Four Community Scenarios

'Between January 1940 and September 1942, 70,723 mental patients were gassed.. chosen by 9 leading professors of psychiatry and 39 top physicians.' Roy Porter, *'Madness, a Brief History.'*

Faulty genetics, environment and life events are all causal factors of mental illness. So too are the stresses of modern life; relationships, work, illness and living in communities. For the human animal, life in communities involves more tolerance, understanding and caring than most people are prepared to give.

Socially inclined animals fight not only at breeding time but also during times of stress for the pack. Unfortunately, it is in human nature to 'fight' those who appear different. What is shocking is when those you least expect so-called civilised people to act in an abhorrent manner. That is the point Roy Porter was making in the epigram above. Prolific UK serial killer Harold Shipman, as I mentioned previously, spoke publicly against unkindness toward mental health patients and was believed a good man. A so-called normal citizen threatened to shoot a young mental patient who was about to be housed next door to him. I have witnessed mental patients show more tolerance and empathy towards neighbours than they received.

Imagine what it might be like to suffer delusions and persecutory voices. As you recover you realize those around you have been mocking you or showing lack of respect. Imagine yourself under such conditions. Might this deepen your illness?

Education
Early attitudes developed because the fickle public tend to think of mental illness only when reading sensational headlines. This gave mentally ill people a negative image. Educational programmes are now carried out in schools and the public are better informed than they

were at the time of the Care in the Community Act. However those with active mental illness rarely receive the same level of empathy offered cancer victims, children with terminal illnesses or someone with an 'acceptable' disability (if such a thing exists). There is a commonly-believed stigma that mental illness is the sufferer's fault. The days when someone with depression is told 'pull your self together' or that depression is a 'moral weakness' is not over, although as this diagnosis spreads, the attitude is gradually changing.

To conclude, better education about mental illness, the work of mental health charities, publications, negotiations with the media over reducing sensationalist headlines, an increasing tendency to present mental illness sympathetically on television, film and radio and lastly recognition of the fact mental illness can affect anyone have lead to a generally more enlightened attitudes in recent times.

East and West

Western medicine is different to Chinese medicine. Eastern cultures retain their past experience, rather than replace old with new as we do in the West. Eastern medicine is steeped in tradition whilst in the West sweeping changes occur with the latest new fad.

Eastern medicine is linked to spirituality in a way increasingly adopted in the West. Whereas Church and belief became almost defunct after the Victorian age, in other cultures it continues to be a bed rock for millions for whom spirituality, daily life, food, exercise and herbal medicine are inextricably linked. The current penchant for holistic therapies borrows much from Eastern traditions offering patients access to a richer mix of therapies.

Evidence Based Treatments

The danger of demand by the Government for evidence-based treatment can threaten this mix. Though evidence-based medicine prevents quackery it can also limit diversity. Few complementary therapies have been through the rigorous system of Government body NICE (National Institute for Clinical Excellence) whose job it is to test medical interventions.

Although laboratory evidence is vital for all pharmaceutical drugs and botanicals (herbal medicines) which have a strong effect on the nervous system, a relaxed approach might be extended to those therapies with anecdotal evidence of effectiveness. Acupuncturists and chiropractors have been deemed acceptable by the medical establishment, but only after a long fight for recognition.

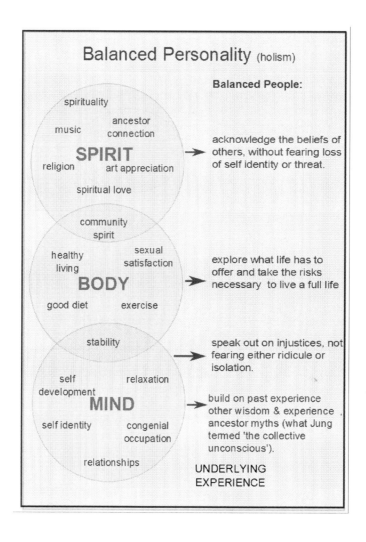

Balanced Personality (holism)

Balanced People:

spirituality

music   ancestor
         connection

SPIRIT   acknowledge the beliefs of
              others, without fearing loss
religion   art appreciation   of self identity or threat.

spiritual love

community
spirit

healthy   sexual
living   satisfaction   explore what life has to
                           offer and take the risks
BODY   necessary to live a full life

good diet   exercise

stability   speak out on injustices, not
             fearing either ridicule or
             isolation.

self   relaxation
development
MIND   build on past experience
                          other wisdom & experience
self identity   congenial   ancestor myths (what Jung
                 occupation   termed 'the collective
                               unconscious').
relationships
                 UNDERLYING
                 EXPERIENCE

Spiritual and non medical treatments are researched through social ('qualitative') methods which allow for anecdotal evidence of success. The 'placebo effect' where Doctors treat anxious patients with inert drugs and 'bedside manner' are proven to work. Some years ago Professor Cathy Sykes of the University of Bristol enquired into the effectiveness of alternative medicines including healing and acupuncture. Dr Sykes holds the Collier Chair in Public Understanding of Science and is known as the 'People's Scientist'. Dr Sykes is working towards a bridge between medicine and alternative therapies. In the BBC documentary series *Alternative Medicine: The Evidence*, she investigated acupuncture, spiritual healing and meditation. Although her views are opposed by some of the scientific community, Dr Sykes believes there is much to be learned. She is interested in links between placebo and faith in spiritual healing.

Professor Sykes' considers the brain far more plastic (adaptable) than is usually considered. This includes the perception of pain. Brain scan readouts have proved how certain acupuncture points markedly affect the area of the brain which deals with the perception of pain. This evidence shows we are still at an early stage in understanding the phenomena of healing. Whilst certain treatments are effective, it is not known why or how. For example, no one knows how ECT works but in 50% of cases it does. Neither is there clinical evidence for all the botanic materials used effectively for centuries as medication. Indeed, plants are the basis of a large number of modern pharmaceutical drugs. Useful plant components continue to be isolated and synthesized for the development of new drugs. Bringing scientific principles to treatment can only be to the good. But this should not prevent acceptance of anecdotal evidence. The balancing factor is charlatanism for personal gain which has always dogged the treatment of mental, as well as physical, illness.

Stress of Living in Communities

Living in communities is a stressful with its indignities, misunderstandings and rebuttals. What we call bullying is known to result in psychiatric injury requiring long term treatment. If community living comes with this negative side, why do we continue to seek out others? It is because we, as descendants of the great apes, are social creatures. Enforced isolation is against our nature.

In a cruel 1950's experiment, psychologists deprived young chimpanzees of their mothers. The young chimps became distressed and some died, proving social shock affects the nervous system.

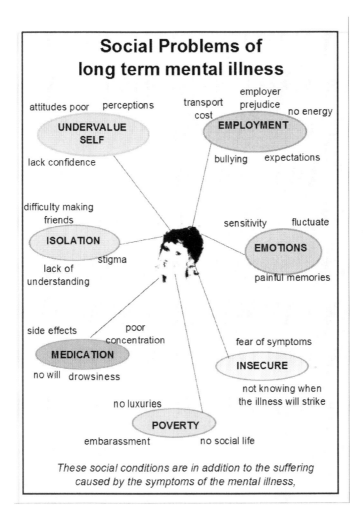

Social Problems of long term mental illness

attitudes poor   perceptions   transport   employer prejudice   no energy
cost

UNDERVALUE SELF   **EMPLOYMENT**

lack confidence   bullying   expectations

difficulty making friends

ISOLATION   sensitivity   fluctuate

stigma   **EMOTIONS**
lack of
understanding   painful memories

side effects   poor
concentration   fear of symptoms

MEDICATION   **INSECURE**

no will   drowsiness   not knowing when
the illness will strike
no luxuries

POVERTY

embarassment   no social life

These social conditions are in addition to the suffering
caused by the symptoms of the mental illness,

In totalitarian states, isolation is still used as a method of torture. Solitary confinement with enforced psychiatric medication leads to mental illness. If exiles are returned to their communities, they suffer extreme anxiety, mistrust and negative symptoms which may last a lifetime. Russian poet Marina Tsvetaeva hanged herself after being isolated for years in appalling conditions in the Russian Gulag. She was aware that her daughter, sister and husband had all been similarly imprisoned. For her, the stress was unbearable and so a gifted poet was in effect murdered and her talent lost to the world.

On the other side, we all know of individuals born into loving families, with a circle of friends and good careers, who succumb to suicide. Mental suffering is insidious because it cannot be seen from the outside, in the way that physical hurts can. Suffering can easily be hidden under smiles and success. We have only to remember Robin Williams, outwardly the clown, but inwardly reaching a level of despair that was shockingly invisible to those who might have helped, had they known.

There is little anyone can do after the event, except acknowledge the seriousness of depressive illness and try to address causal factors. As well as individual and family support, mental wellbeing is associated with living and belonging to a thriving community. I offer four examples to demonstrate this theme.

Four Community Scenarios

What would happen in your community to these individuals:

- a woman sees people no one else sees or hears.
- a man mutters in the street, scratching his head until it bleeds.
- a female child is heard screaming and crying at night

Refer to the diagram on the next page, which shows reactions in four fictitious communities.

In community A All are recognized as behaving strangely, but the community is compassionate. The woman is sent for observation to a psychiatric hospital. The man is offered social support and treatment. The child is taken into care when it is discovered she is the victim of parental abuse.

In community B Ancestors are revered. All three are looked upon with awe as they are believed to have the spirits of deceased tribe members, and are well treated. Their families are given gifts.

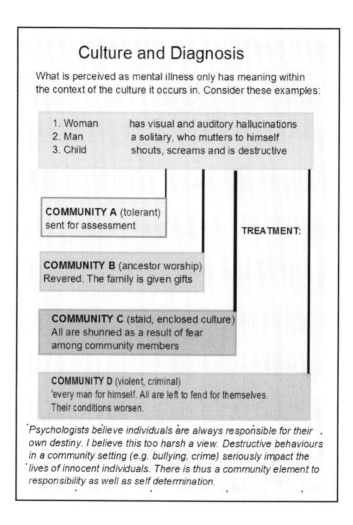

Culture and Diagnosis

What is perceived as mental illness only has meaning within the context of the culture it occurs in. Consider these examples:

1. Woman — has visual and auditory hallucinations
2. Man — a solitary, who mutters to himself
3. Child — shouts, screams and is destructive

COMMUNITY A (tolerant)
sent for assessment

TREATMENT:

COMMUNITY B (ancestor worship)
Revered. The family is given gifts

COMMUNITY C (staid, enclosed culture)
All are shunned as a result of fear among community members

COMMUNITY D (violent, criminal)
'every man for himself. All are left to fend for themselves. Their conditions worsen.

Psychologists believe individuals are always responsible for their own destiny. I believe this too harsh a view. Destructive behaviours in a community setting (e.g. bullying, crime) seriously impact the lives of innocent individuals. There is thus a community element to responsibility as well as self determination.

The community would be outraged if it was suggested any of them were mentally ill and the individuals are cared for by the whole community.

In community C People are afraid of strange behaviour which is believed to stem from bad spirits. The woman is hanged, the man exiled, the child tortured then murdered.

In community D There is a history of violence and crime. The three go unnoticed. The woman becomes ill and stabs a man under the delusion he is attacking her. The man is followed by a gang of youths who taunt him. He commits suicide. The child is hit by her parents. She runs away and is found by a pimp (someone who lives off the earnings of prostitutes). He drugs her and forces her into prostitution. She is found dead in a squalid bedsit, a syringe by her side.

Although the characters and communities are fictitious, they are based on real life circumstances. Sometimes it is not a matter of where you live but the society you are born into which determines your fate if you have a mental condition. If you can cope with difficult subject matter read the *Victoria Climbie Enquiry* which details the horrific murder of a small child whose relatives believed she was a witch. More horrific is the fact her murder took place not in a remote part of the third world - but in London.

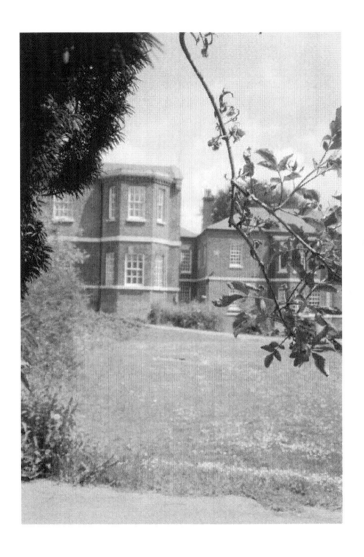

Chapter 3
Mental Illness to 17th Century

Content:
Bethlem Asylum –Medieval to 17th Century
Primitive Beliefs
Historic Trepanning
Ancient Civilizations
Hippocrates and Medical Reasoning
Other Ancient Treatments
Medieval Belief
Bethlehem Hospital
16th Century – Change of Attitude
Lazar Houses Revamped as Asylums
Ship of Fools
Bethlem Asylum – Medieval to 17th Century

The perceived cause of mental illness has a strong bearing on how the illness is perceived by society. The kind of treatment offered (or not) very much depends upon that factor (see examples in previous chapter). It is a useful and interesting exercise to look at the history of mental illness with this in view. There are many books on the subject but I recommend Roy Porter (see further resources).

Primitive Beliefs
Although no one will ever know for certain how early man thought, Archaeologists make educated guesses through examining artefacts and structures at grave sites, comparing them with similar sites world wide. Apart from decorative art, it is commonly accepted that primitive people drew pictures on cave walls as acts of faith which created the right conditions for successful hunting. Sacrificial victims have been found with all manner of injuries; from burning, hanging, bludgeoning, beheading, to living organs cut out. Although civilised people view such sacrifices as repugnant, they make sense in terms of the primitive mindset. If you were terrified of powerful gods who sent storms, eclipse, or crop failure if not offered appeasement, and sacrifice was accepted in your community, you either did the same or took the consequences.

Whilst belief in gods led to horrific acts by modern standards it also lead to the building of stupendous monuments, such as Stonehenge, still regarded with awe thousands of years later.

Historic Trepanning

Not all primitive magic was aimed at warding off death and natural destruction. In the pre-medical age, Shamans or ritual priests were responsible for healing. Evidence has been found of a type of crude brain surgery in 40,000 year old skulls. Circular holes found in skulls in the Neolithic age are assumed to be a practice that let out evil spirits. This primitive surgery has echoes in many ancient cultures - Stone Age, Ancient Greece and Rome. Surprisingly, there is evidence of bone growth around the holes, proving some of the patients survived the operation. Trepanning, using an electric drill, is still practiced by modern surgeons, albeit rarely, to relieve pressure where head wounds have left the brain pressing on the skull.

Ancient Civilizations

Man began worshipping gods to seek favours or to relieve afflictions of mind and body. The gods were believed to be powerful creatures who punished disobedient humans. As men began living in larger communities, the god culture underwent changes. Rather than individuals offering sacrifice, powerful men interceded with gods on behalf of the community, as well as acting as healers. These were shamans or priests and held considerable power and wealth. Priests were the forerunners of physicians and we assume it was these people who carried out the trepanning.

The ancient Greeks were fond of philosophy and developed a sophisticated belief system about deities. Their gods punished any opposition by meting out moral tasks. Below is a simplified version of an ancient Greek tragedy. When you read it, keep in mind the twin Greek beliefs:

- disobeying a god is punishable by the Furies
- matricide (killing a mother) is punishable by death

Myth of the House of Agamemnon

The god Apollo orders Orestes, son of King Agamemnon & Queen Clytemnestra, to put his mother to death because she and her lover Aegisthus had murdered her husband. Orestes agonises over the god's direction. If he kills Clytemnestra he disobeys goddess Athena's law (i.e. that matricide is punishable by death). If he refuses, he will be disobeying Apollo and be hounded by the Furies. Orestes aided by his sister Elektra, kills Clytemnestra and her lover. Orestes is then inflicted with madness by the Furies. Just as Orestes is nearing the point of death, Athena forgives him and the curse is lifted.

The Greeks were fond of moral dramas. These were plays featuring masked players and a Chorus of actors representing the voices of conscience. None of these dramas end happily. The hero or heroine inevitably dies or is sent mad. It is the ancient equivalent of *The Terminator*. Centuries before Sigmund Freud, the Greeks had recognized that moral dilemmas (mental conflict) could result in loss of reason. Once the conflicts had been worked through, the sufferer was cleansed and would recover. This is not too far from Freudian thinking - or even modern drama therapy.

When animal sacrifices or moral retribution no longer appeared enough to appease unhappy and vindictive gods, hey presto - the scapegoat was invented. Scapegoats were chosen to do all the suffering for tribes or communities. The scapegoat was at first literally a goat or chicken, but might also be a bull or a human – or animal and human for greater effect. A scapegoat had several purposes:

- to appease the deity, so the victim got off or was cured
- to provide the deity with a gift
- to allow a community to 'get off' any punishment

Of course, certain communities or individuals could easily seize the opportunity of making a 'scapegoat' of something they envied or wanted to eliminate. This is comparable to the witch hunts I mentioned earlier, or modern 'scapegoating' of politicians, bankers, lawyers or other unpopular 'trades'. This is an example of a scapegoat:

Office scapegoat: In an organisation, major changes are made which affect existing staff. The staff fear expressing opposition to the plans, because they do not want to be seen as trouble makers. There is a tense atmosphere. Someone who does not fit in, is different, timid or perhaps envied becomes the focus for all the ensuing problems and is ejected. For a short time, until the next 'issue', all goes quiet, which seems to 'prove' the scapegoat was indeed to blame. Those who threw spanners in the works experience the double delight of getting rid of their rivals without punishment. Bystanders are relieved it was *'not their fault'*. Managers are relieved the issue has been resolved.

Scapegoat System

Early humans believed powerful Deities controlled nature. Communities appeased them by offering animal sacrifices.

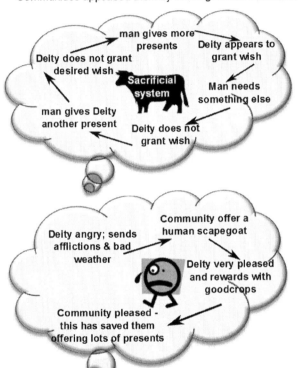

The scapegoat is personalised. Something goes wrong & it is assumed a Deity is displeased with someone. An individual is killed to represent the sorrow of the community. The Deity is 'appeased'.

The triangle of sin/ punishment / sacrifice can be understood as antecedents of **moral panics** explained earlier.

Hippocrates and Medical Reasoning

Hippocrates was a Greek philosopher who was highly regarded in his day and now credited as the father of modern medicine. He made the first study of mental illness, nearly two thousand years ago. Hippocrates disagreed with conventional views and concluded madness was *'no more divine nor sacred than other diseases but has a natural cause.'* Hippocrates overturned the Greek view of madness as punishment by gods. Pre-empting the practices of modern science he used examination of patients and observation to isolate three types of mental disorder:

- brain fever
- mania
- melancholia

These terms remained in use until the nineteenth century. The term mania is still used. Shakespeare accurately describes melancholia or what is now called depressive illness in his play Hamlet. Hippocrates, Galen and their followers made a study of the four humors or vital fluids. The Greeks believed if the vital fluids were not in harmony, this would lead to illness [see following diagram]. This belief is closely allied with Chinese medicine and Western alternative therapies.

There is a parallel in modern psychiatry, in that depression is believed to be an imbalance of natural brain chemicals.

I depict this crossover in belief of early medicine, science, philosophy and nature in the form of a Mandela [next page]. Mandelas represent balancing forces and circular in form. Mandelas were used in magic rituals. Starting from the outer circle are:

- alchemy - elemental symbols air, earth, fire, water
- seasons – each fixed with certain religious rites
- physical states - caused by imbalance of humours
- humours –vital body fluids

In the sixteenth century, an Apothecary would treat patients by 'balancing' the humours, using lancets, blood letting or leeches:

- purging – through inducing vomiting
- bloodletting - using lancets or leeches
- inducing fever or cold, according to the malady

Unfortunately purging often killed patients, as did the application of leeches and bleeding, yet this did not prevent this form of treatment continuing into the 18th and 19th centuries. In a retrospective, 21st century surgeons began using leeches to clean infected wounds, finding them more effective and less harmful than strong medications. Leeches secrete a solution which prevents blood clotting and can be coaxed into difficult-to-reach areas of the body. As modern patients find leeches repugnant, practitioners resorted to hiding the leech in a coloured plastic shield.

Other Ancient Treatments

The Greek philosopher Plato wrote that 'madmen' ought to be locked away at home. The term did not have the same pejorative meaning it holds today. This practice of locking away was widespread until the early nineteenth century. Romans were familiar with depression, which they called melancholy. They treated this illness with warm baths, music and well-lit rooms. Such treatments would still be considered beneficial.

Greeks and Romans used sleep temples with soporific herbs given as curatives to aid rest and sleep. In modern times *modified narcosis* was used with depressed patients exhausted through lack of sleep. The narcosis was induced by drugs.

Romans reportedly used electric eels to shock patients out of madness. In 19th century Bethlem Hospital patients were lowered into a tub of eels for the same purpose. This curious treatment may be a precursor of electric shock treatment (ECT).

Medieval Belief

In medieval times, mental illness was attributed to divine retribution or witchcraft. But, surprisingly, there was also a more enlightened attitude towards those identified as *idiots* or *lunatics* (again, these terms did not have the prejudicial connotation they have today); by idiot they meant, born defective; lunatic meant afflicted by the moon.

Belief in witchcraft lasted until late into the 17th century. Sick people and animals were believed possessed by evil spirits as a result of curses made by witches (human servants of the devil). The Church, concerned at immoral sexual activity between monks and nuns, blamed the Devil for inciting them to passion. The Devils of Loudun by Aldous Huxley (and the film of the same name directed by Ken Russell) is a graphic depiction of this story.

Mandela

Throughout the ages, circular symmetries (mandelas) were believed to have magical and healing properties. This diagram illustrates mandelas from nature, alchemy and early medicine.

Illness was believed caused by imbalances in the vital fluids (humours). Doctors treated patients by 're-balancing' these fluids - using leeches (blood letting), induced fever or cold. Thus, symmetry was restored and the patient recovered.

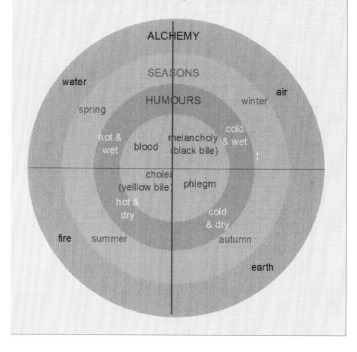

In contrast is a rare and interesting case cited by David and Christine Roffe in the British Medical Journal. Emma de Beston was a medieval woman brought before a local Inquisition to be examined for lunacy. The woman was treated fairly by the Inquisition, who saw through the wicked intent of relatives, who were trying to deprive her of liberty and property. Although she did not recover her reason, the Inquisition enabled her to regain her property and access welfare. This case is a model which Roffe compares with less favourable patient experiences of the Care in the Community Act (1990's).

Bethlehem Hospital

Bethlehem (Bethlem or Bedlam) was an insane Asylum set up through public subscription in 1377. It was on the site of the much earlier Priory the Church of St Mary of Bethlehem. The first mentally ill patients were recorded in 1403 when it also housed poor and physically ill patients.

Private *madhouses* were run as businesses by Physicians. Wealthy patients paid for their keep and quack medicines, whilst fees for the poor were funded by the Parish. Previously, those deemed insane had been prosecuted and imprisoned for bizarre or anti-social behaviour. Bethlem was an alternative to prison, though whether the patients were better off is doubtful. Bethlem kept the insane out of harm's way but more pertinently removed them from the sight of family and society. Asylums quickly became dumping grounds for unwanted relatives or misfits. In this age there was no distinction between physical and mental illness, nor between social or forensic (criminal) cases. An Asylum housed anyone not deemed fit to live in society:

• organic brain disease – epilepsy, cerebral palsy
• head injuries
• socially unacceptable - prostitutes, thieves, beggars
• anyone deemed a lunatic or simple (historic terms)

16th Century – Change of Attitude

By the 16th Century mental illness came to be seen as an illness or malady and not divine punishment, that is, they believed that the illness could be treated. Roy Porter describes the changing view quoting philosopher Descartes *'reason can rescue man from insanity'*. Nevertheless, becoming mad was considered to be something only curable through prayer and bible reading. This view helped the church maintain power over frightened communities. Later in the century, monasteries and nunneries began to provide shelter for the insane within their communities and inmates were treated kindly.

Lazar Houses Revamped as Asylums

In his excellent book *Madness and Civilization* (1960's) Michel Foucault makes interesting parallels between religious fervour and the exclusion of those perceived as sinners. Leprosy had been a scourge from the Middle Ages and thousands of Lazar Houses had been set up to offer lepers' refuge, after they had been forcibly excluded from communities. Popular belief dictated that leprosy was a punishment for sins and to cast out a leper was seen as an act of religious piety. As Foucault ironically remarks '*the sinner who abandons the leper at his door opens his* [the sinner's] *way to heaven*'.

By the 16th Century this policy of social exclusion had a knock-on beneficial outcome. By separating lepers from society, the spread of leprosy reduced, because the disease is spread through contact. By the end of the century, Lazar Houses were almost emptied. The crumbling buildings were re-used to isolate those considered outcasts.

Ship of Fools

There was another convenient way of tidying the streets. There was a supposed affinity between calmness and the sea, it being a common belief the sea would cure mad minds. Foucault describes madmen being given into the care of mariners, who took them on long voyages in trading ships. Some of these lunatic travellers did improve because of the better environment; being removed from public humiliation, accessing fresh air, fresh food and calm. But other unfortunates died lonely deaths far from their native country. No doubt some were put over the side if mariners could not cope with their behaviour. Casting humans overboard alive was common during the slave trade. *Ship of Fools* became an allegorical term in both its romantic and macabre aspects, written into folklore and art. Read Foucault's splendid book for more detail.

Bethlem Asylum – Medieval to 17th Century

It is ironic that ancient Rome provided Temples of Sleep with light and air for people in mental turmoil, whilst up to the 18th century incarceration in grim Asylums was commonplace. Mental symptoms were feared or laughed at and considered incurable. When Bethlem Hospital opened, none of its inhabitants were expected to recover. Most died within its grim walls after decades of malnourishment and maltreatment. Male and female patients were kept in appalling

31

conditions, naked, restrained or chained, sleeping on straw bedding. Vomiting and purging were thought to reduce a patient's strength in order to control them. It was considered wasteful to feed patients too much in view of purging. The following are 17th century Bethlem treatments, with the beliefs that inspired them. Patients were:

- put in a tub with electric eels [shock them to wellness]
- subject to blood letting [excess blood causes madness]
- put into water in a box with holes [fear forced a patient to sanity]
- spinning patient on a stool [shaking the brain into sanity]
- cutting off the clitoris [sexual organs caused melancholia]

Physicians in Bethlem formulated quack medicines, which patients had to pay for. This gave the Physicians handsome profits. On Sundays, people could pay 1d to view patients as an entertainment but visitors interested in patient welfare were discouraged. In 1770 this noxious practice was banned. 17th century artist William Hogarth famous series The Rake's Progress accurately portrayed a scene in Bethlem. Occasionally patients were discharged and given a badge as a license to beg in surrounding villages. In a cruel reversal, they were expected to repay the cost of their treatment in Bethlem out of their meagre earnings.

As a matter of interest, Bethlem hospital has a museum containing the art of mentally ill people from Victorian times and is open to the public on certain days.

Chapter 4
Mental Illness to 20th Century

Content:
The York Retreat 1796
Degeneration (Benedict Morel 1809 – 1873)
Asylums after 1820
Victorian Poets and Fashionable Melancholia
Psychosurgery
Hypnosis, & Psychology (Charcot, Breuer, Freud & Jung)
Behaviourists (Pavlov, Watson, Thorndike & Skinner
Asylums in the 20th Century
1950's Lithium Valium and Largactil
Token Economy
1960's – 1970's Encounter Groups
Cognitive Behavioural Therapies
Milton Erickson 1970's
2000 Anti Psychiatric Movement: Szaz & Laing
Dialectical Behaviour Therapy (DBT)
Cognitive Therapies
21st Century – Virtual Brain Simulation
Psychopathic Personality Disorder and the Law
Therapeutic Relationship
Neuro-Typical v Non Neuro-typical

By the early eighteenth century madness was viewed as a disease of the mind, although little was known about its cause or treatment.

In 1788 King George III was diagnosed with mental illness and was locked away during his florid episodes. Doctors treated him with antimony which contains arsenic, which most likely worsened to his illness. He was treated cruelly by his Physicians, being chained in a straightjacket, gagged and treated with cupping, a painful procedure which resulted in festering sores. King George is now believed to have contracted porphyria through ingestion of arsenic used to powder his wigs and excessive antimony prescribed by Physicians.

During the 18th century, Physicians started to explore links between the nervous system, senses and intellect. Studies were made of shaking palsy (epilepsy), tics, hallucinations and aphasia (disturbance of the senses). Phrenology was briefly popular before being discredited.

Phrenology was invented by two anatomists, who were convinced that the shape of specific parts of the head reflected the personality.

The York Retreat 1796

In 1796, Quaker William Tuke set up an institution based on moral therapy. All the patients lived-in, learning social skills from staff. Tuke had witnessed a fellow Quaker dying in an Asylum and was determined no-one else should suffer in this way. His patients were rewarded for good behaviour and punished for bad - a moral / bible therapy. The Retreat is still active though not in its original form. It was a forerunner of modern sanctuaries like Maytree in London, where suicidal patients can stay up to four days in a quiet environment with access to therapists.

Degeneration (Benedict Morel 1809 – 1873)

The nineteenth century brought huge interest in the treatment of mental illness with many new theories. Morel believed that defects in families degenerated down the generations. He outlined the stages as:

1. alcohol and opiate addiction
2. prostitution and sexual degeneracy
3. criminality
4. insanity
5. imbecility {historic term}
6. sterility [end of the family line]

There was no classification for distinguishing between forensic, mental illness, organic mental disorders, learning difficulties or any other neurological phenomena, all mental disorders being classed the same. Morel believed *degeneracy* or reversal was caused by drug or alcohol abuse, diseases such as malaria or moral sickness. He believed diseased families would die out naturally over time.

There is a sort of loose parallel with Darwin's early theories of natural selection and of gene theory. However, Morel's theories spawned the quasi -science of eugenics, disastrously adopted by the Nazis to exterminate the Jewish race.

Asylums after 1820

A Victorian Asylum held up to 1000 patients in its own community. Asylums were built on sites with a large amount of land, with room for a large number of support buildings such as kitchens, chapels, laundries, industrial units and kitchen gardens.

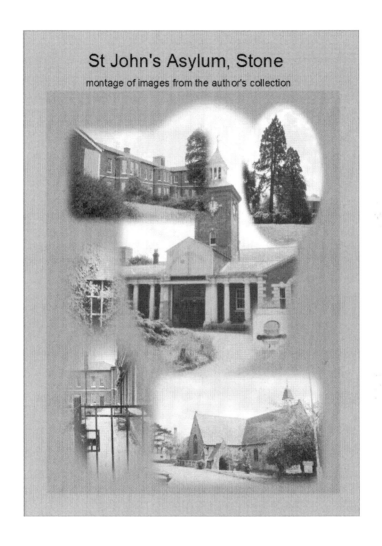

Patients had to take up a trade such as shoe-making, laundry work or gardening. They were expected to work as hard as their peers in the infamous Workhouses. Asylums were not seen as places of recuperation but houses of moral correction. The saving grace was the countryside locations with clean air, fresh vegetables and their distance from mocking townsfolk.

Asylums were initially administered by Superintendents. These were men, not medically qualified but experienced in dealing with the bizarre and often violent inmate behaviour. This was in pre medication days, when there were no effective ways of reducing the symptoms and behaviours of psychosis. An 1820 Act of Parliament made it compulsory to have medically qualified practitioners in attendance and for regular inspections.

By 1845 every county had to build an Asylum by law. By 1890 two medical certificates had to be signed before anyone could be detained. These measures were brought in to stem cruel practices like dumping unwanted relatives or wives, for life, in Asylums.

Socially unacceptable relatives (historic term: moral defectives) in Asylums when these people had no symptoms of mental illness. There were also those who sought early inheritance by locking away unwanted relatives. Many Victorian creatives were incarcerated in Asylums, including artist Richard Dadd and poet William Cowper. Rich patients were treated either in private madhouses run by Doctors or in their own homes. However, there were kinder institutions.

Reformer Robert Gardiner Hill ran the Lincoln Asylum where restraints were replaced with activity-centred therapy, wholesome diet, exercises and art therapy. Not surprisingly such regimes proved successful.

If you want to see what Asylums look like, try your local Records Office. My monochrome images of St John's Asylum, Stone, near Aylesbury are held in the archives of the Centre for Buckinghamshire Studies. There is a montage on the previous page.

Victorian Poets and Fashionable Melancholia

Victorians created an enduring romantic image of pale and languid artistic types sitting among idyllic sylvan scenes whilst partaking of laudanum (opium and brandy) to enhance their writing. Self induced melancholia was popular with Keats, Shelley, Byron, Dickens,

Coleridge and abolitionist William Wilberforce. The 'mildly mad' popular Victorian image was attached to Lord Byron who was famously referred to by his lover, Lady Caroline Lamb, as '*mad, bad and dangerous to know*'.

The truth was less delightful. There were frequent deaths from arsenic or laudanum taken to get the popular 'tuberculosis look'; pallid flesh and large eyes - similar to the look adopted by 21st century Goths. The melancholia exhibited by these socialites was far from the truth of depressive illness and suicidal, frequently brought about by excessive consumption of cheap gin. Hogarth's engraving Gin Lane depicts such a scene.

Psychosurgery
Phineas Gage

In 1848 an event took place which radically altered the treatment of behaviour disorders. Railroad worker Phineas Gage was exploding rocks with dynamite when a charge went off accidentally, driving a long 25mm diameter steel rod up into his brain through his eye. Immediately after this horrific accident Gage became unconscious, suffering fits. Although he survived for 11 years after the accident his personality underwent a change and he became so aggressive his friends said they no longer recognised him. Gage was studied by many eminent physicians of his day. He died of a series of seizures nearly a decade after the accident.

Gage's skull is in the Warren Anatomical Museum of Harvard Medical School. Recently, photographs of Gage have been identified and these can be viewed online. Gage's brain was examined by scientists and as a result of this research they located the area of brain affecting personality and mood.

Pre-Frontal Leucotomy

Modern brain surgery began as a result of research on Gage's brain. Surgeons experimented with a procedure called lobotomy (or leucotomy) in which the frontal lobes of the brain are severed. The hope was to find a cure for schizophrenia and chronic depression which would not respond to other treatments. The first lobotomy was carried out by Egas Moniz in 1935. He won the 1949 Nobel Prize for his work. Moniz was shot dead by a patient he had lobotomised.

Psychiatrist Walter Freeman carried out over 2000 lobotomy operations, sweeping an ice pick under the brow-ridge of his patients. 50,000 patients underwent such operations in the 1950's and 10% died. This crude surgery was always controversial even among

Psychiatrists. Some believed that interfering with personality through surgery was unethical. These operations had a bad effect on personality, mood and social functioning and were irreversible. Lobotomy was discontinued in 1975. I met one of the last lobotomised patients whilst working in a Scottish Asylum in the late 1970's. She had been, according to medical reports, a normal and intelligent young woman, but after the operation she wandered the locked Ward she lived in, constantly crying and having lost her capacity to reason.

Hypnosis & Psychology (Charcot, Breuer, Freud & Jung)
Charcot [1835 - 1893] & Breuer [1842 - 1925]
Hypnotherapy is the grandfather of the psychotherapies. Jean Martin Charcot, its inventor, worked extensively with patients diagnosed with hysterical paralyses of limb or voice, now called *conversion disorders* (paralyses as a result of psychological trauma). Conversion disorders were common in the early eighteenth century. Charcot discovered a deep form of relaxation he called hypnosis. He used hypnotic suggestion to successfully free patients from physical symptoms. Charcot did not know how his treatment worked, but it did.

Following on from his work, Charcot's colleague Joseph Breuer allowed patients to talk under hypnosis. The term 'talking cure' was coined by Breuer's celebrated cases Anna O, who used it to describe how she was freed from neurotic symptoms after being hypnotised.

Sigmund Freud [1856 1939]
Freud was a devotee of Charcot and Breuer and collaborated with both men during his early career. Breuer and Freud coined a new term *catharsis* (Greek for cleansing or discharging) to describe the process of treatment. Freud developed a theory of mind over a number of years, after studying the action of catharsis in his patients. It is unfortunate that while Freud became internationally famous, the pioneering work of Charcot and Breuer have became largely forgotten.

Freud developed psychoanalysis from hypnosis. His life work was studying the hidden world of mind or subconscious. As an aside, the location of 'mind' within the brain remains unknown.

Freud came to believe that the hypnotic state was not responsible for cure but the therapeutic relationship between doctor and patient. He discarded hypnosis, allowing his patients to talk freely in the conscious state. Freud used dream analysis to gain access to the subconscious. He referred to dreams as, *'the royal road to the unconscious'*; that is, a way of interpreting the unconscious mind. He encouraged patients to analyse the meaning of the symbolic language in their dreams.

Another method Freud used was *free association*. The patient was encouraged to say anything which came into their mind. This, he believed, triggered hidden memories repressed by the conscious mind. Through re-visiting and gaining insight (understanding) into painful earlier experiences, Freud's patients became psychologically healthier and had better relationships.

A great deal of negative publicity surrounded Freud's early theory that children had repressed sexual fantasies about their parents. Freud came to believe that children only matured when they were able to accept they could not have a sexual relationship with their parent. He believed *rape fantasy* was an expression of their unconscious wish to mate with their parents. This rape fantasy theory negatively affected children who had been raped by a parent and were not believed. This belief unfortunately existed for generations, until Freud himself renounced his theory. However, this cannot negate the contribution Freud made to understanding the nature of mind. Freud and his follower Carl Jung were the founding fathers of psychology.

Carl Jung [1875 - 1961] - Analytical Psychology

Jung was a devotee of Freud. Freud expected Jung to become his heir and continue supporting psychoanalytic theory. But Jung began to have doubts and eventually split with his mentor to formulate his own theories. Jung was deeply interested in philosophy, mythology, spiritual and religious beliefs.

Jung made a study of the Pueblo Indian tribe who believed their rituals made the sun move around the sky, ensuring continuity of the seasons. This belief, that they were integral to the cycle of existence, gave Pueblo Indians a strong sense of confidence. Jung concluded it was essential for everyone to include a spiritual dimension in their life and that this would strengthen their psyche.

From his extensive studies in world mythology, Jung discovered links between cultures and across generations. He noticed that many character types reoccurred and gave these names, such as hero, wise man, mother, fool. Each of these types had a particular life journey. The hero's journey - a man is born of a virgin and sacrificed by his people, then he is resurrected and returns to save them.

For further reading, try:

- Larousse Book of World Mythology
- Standard Stories from the Opera
- Man and his Symbols (Jung)

Jung discovered that *personality* is a process of the mind and it is made up of many archetypical types. The work of a Jungian Analyst is to assist the patient to integrate their *archetypes* in a process Jung termed *individuation*. Refer to the diagram on the next page.

Jung's studies of archetypes lead to his consideration of the carrier which allowed memories to be retained through generations. His solution was the *collective unconscious*. Archetypal memories lie in the unconscious but can be triggered into the conscious under certain conditions:

- the symbolism of dreams
- déjà vue – feeling something has been experienced before
- memories – memories not connected with direct experience

Déjà vue is an interesting phenomenon which is depicted in the movie *Groundhog Day*. Déjà vue may be connected with *false memory syndrome* where people insist they have experienced something which could not have happened.

Jung also coined the terms:

- introvert - inner reflective personality
- extrovert - worldly and sociable personality

Jung carried out his studies decades before scientists developed genetic theory. If you consider his conclusions in this light, his work is remarkable. Sadly he wrote few books to explain his theories or how they might be integrated, - a work left to his followers.

Behaviourists (Pavlov, Watson, Thorndike & Skinner)

Behaviourists were psychologists seeking rational explanations for human behaviour. Renowned behaviourists are:

- Ivan Pavlov [1849 -1936]
- John Watson [1878-1958]
- Edward Thorndike [1874-1949]
- Burrus Skinner [1904 - 1990]

Conscious & Unconscious Mind
ways of processing experience

Some scientists believe mind exists in all sensory cells, not just the brain.

4. Output thinking (conscious)

We form conclusions about experiences from the products of 1, 2 and 3 - sensory input; comparison with past experience; collective unconscious. This processing determines if the current event (new experience) is viewed in a negative or posiive way.

This accounts for situations when we have a 'gut feeling' that something is positive or negative without consciously knowing why.

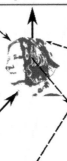

1. Input through the senses - in the conscious mind

we experience events through sight, taste, touch, hearing and smell. These are then processed in short term memory

2. Comparison with unconscious mind (memory)

the event is filtered to a part of memory where it is compared with past experience

3. The collective unconscious

the Collective Unconscious was a theory of Carl Jung; it is the part of mind apparent in dreams or feelings such as 'deja veu' (a sense of having experienced the same even on a previous occasion). The collective unconsioucs contains our cultural and racial myths.

Ivan Pavlov conducted experiments on animal behaviour. Pavlov proved how responses to a stimulus could be changed in animals through a now-famous experiment. Pavlov rang a bell each time his dogs were given food. Before long the dogs started to salivate as soon as they heard the bell, which lead him to conclude it was the bell, and not the food, which had triggered salivation.

Pavlov's collaborator John Watson continued this work in humans, discovering how human behaviour can be conditioned (changed) through life experience. Skinner continued Thorndike's work by placing rats in a maze. The rats were rewarded for going in the right direction and punished by electric shock for going the wrong way. He concluded that animals learn through reward and punishment. Or perhaps rats like an easy life too..

These arguments continue in the great debate of 'nature versus nurture'; whether human behaviour is inborn or due to upbringing and environment. Behavioural therapy was used to treat depressive illness, phobias and addictions.

Asylums in the 20th Century

By the late 20th century Asylums housed very aged patients from the Victorian era, who had been incarcerated virtually all their lives. I met some of the last surviving patients of this social injustice. By now in their 80's/90's they lived out their lives in Asylums, with fellow patients performing the function of friends and family. One patient was an unmarried mother diagnosed as a social misfit. Another had stolen a bicycle as a teenager and been 'put away' by his embarrassed parents, never to return to the community.

To this sad group were added a new tranche of patients with behavioural problems. Symptoms were often bizarre with no psychiatric medication to relieve them. I have already related the story of the Queen's cousins, who were the focus of a 1980 expose in *The Sun* Newspaper and a Channel 4 documentary. To repeat, Katherine and Nerissa Bowes-Lyon were locked in Asylums because they were born with learning disabilities and their parents felt no longer able to care for them. These children were listed in Burkes Peerage as dead in the early 1960's, to avoid embarrassment to the Royal Family. Neither received visits or presents from their illustrious relatives.

New treatments were introduced in the 20th century, including a form of behavioural therapy called *Token Economy* (explained later) and newly invented drugs Largactil and Lithium.

Despite the grim buildings many and varied facilities were set up within the Asylum (now rebranded 'Psychiatric Hospitals'); libraries, shops, Occupational Therapy units, canteens and laundry rooms. The refurbished Asylums had their own chapel and Chaplain. Visits to the local town were frequent and considered part of treatment. Residents of the village remained tolerant of bizarre behaviour because they had grown used to it, even when such behaviours were uncontrolled, due to the lack of effective anti psychotic drugs.

Patients were dressed from a communal pool of clothing, which would not occur nowadays. Beds ranged along each side of an open plan ward. Very few patients had personal possessions or pictures of family and the whole scenario was institutional. They were all woken early, as in a prison, for the round of 'topping and tailing' [dressing and toileting] and breakfast, before the ward rounds during which drugs were administered. Wards were run on authoritarian lines by a Ward Sister. The keynote was efficiency and hygiene. The hygiene might appear excessive by our standards, however it is recognised this was no bad thing, considering the frequent outbreaks of infectious disease in 21st century hospitals.

1950's Lithium Valium and Largactil

After the 1950's, a drug called Lithium was developed to treat mania and manic depressive psychosis (MDP). Lithium is a metal salt which effectively levels mood, but is lethal if overdosed. Patients on this medication had regular blood tests. Early anti-psychotic drugs such as Largactil were clumsy and known as *liquid coshes* because they made patients lethargic. In the 1960's tranquillisers Librium and Valium were prescribed, mainly to neurotic women, until being withdrawn from use when they were found to be addictive. The development of psychiatric medication was at its height throughout these decades up until the 1980's and the brief rise of Prozac. Heralded as the wonder drug and a cure for depression this class of drug (SSRI's) was later damned as a potential causal factor of suicide.

Token Economy

Token economy was a 1970's form of behavioural therapy. Patients were rewarded for good behaviour by being given plastic tokens which they could exchange for cigarettes, cups of tea and treats like biscuits. But human nature always triumphs. What the psychologists on the Ward might not have realized was a black economy in tokens going on late at night after day staff left.

1960's – 1970's Encounter Groups

Encounter groups were based on work by Carl Rogers, Fritz Perls and others who had the idealistic aim of improving human potential. In T Groups and later Encounter Groups members were encouraged to discuss their deepest feelings with other members. However, this was based on a trust system which ultimately did not work because the group leaders were not all they should have been. Vulnerable members of the group were at risk from vociferous others. Encounter Groups are now discredited.

Cognitive Behavioural Therapies

Cognitive (= *to recognise*) therapists believed that those who consistently experienced frustrations, anxieties and emotional problems in life had faulty patterns of thinking. They attributed these negative thinking patterns to dysfunctional childhood or negative life experience.

Cognitive therapy was a psychological approach which helped patients recognize, challenge and change negative thoughts and their associated negative emotions and behaviour.

Behavioural and cognitive therapies were later combined into cognitive-behavioural therapy (CBT) which remains treatment of choice for psychological elements of mental illnesses.

Milton Erickson 1970's

In the 1970's Milton Erickson (an American Psychiatrist) pioneered a method which had patients flocking to his clinics. During his early life Erickson developed polio and was confined to bed. Bored, Erickson started observing his visitors, noting their behaviour and body language. Erickson watched his siblings from the time they crawled to walking stage. From these observations he re-taught himself to walk.

Over several years, Erickson developed his theory of symbolic language; everyone has a unique psychological 'map of the world'. Ericksonian therapy entailed helping the patient discover and utilise their personal map, or inner resources. Erickson would talk to a patient using their unique symbolic language (metaphors). This therapy is comparable to the theories of Freud and Jung, who both analysed the unique symbolism in their patients' dreams.

The crux of Erickson's method was establishing the meaning of the problem from the patient's point of view. Erickson initially advocated auto-hypnosis, where in a very relaxed state the patient was encouraged to imagine themselves free of their problem, describing how life would be without that problem. From that point, Erickson set his patient tasks which were designed to enhance the healing.

Unfortunately, enthusiasts tried to rigidly mimic his methodology including Erickson's hand and body movements. Erickson never intended this. What he advocated was therapists developing their own techniques for treating patients. Erickson's work was taken up by many so-called brief therapists who copied his system without understanding the underlying principles.

2000 Anti Psychiatric Movement: Szaz & Laing

'In psychiatry we use one set of laws to explain sane behaviour which we attribute to reasons (choices) and another set of laws to explain insane behaviour which we attribute to causes (diseases).' Thomas Szaz 2001.

Psychiatrists Thomas Szaz and R D Laing held the controversial view that mental illness was a construct of society and had no other meaning for the patient. Laing believed psychoses should not be treated with drug therapy. This is recognised as detrimental; untreated psychoses cause unnecessary suffering and prolonging trauma.

The anti-psychiatric movement grew as service users (people who use mental health services), frustrated with the side effects of drugs and lack of effective treatments, sought other solutions. The anti-psychiatry books by Szaz, Laing and their followers make interesting reading in the light of 21st century patient preference for talking or complementary therapies. However there are certain mind states like psychosis which Psychiatrists always treat with drug therapy, until something more effective is discovered.

Dialectical Behaviour Therapy (DBT)

Dialectical behaviour therapy (DBT) was developed out of CBT by American Psychologist Dr Marsha Lineham and was used for treating personality disorders and crippling emotional problems. Dialectical means at either end. The name reflects both ends of high emotional states experienced by people with personality disorders. Patients who undergo DBT are likely to have felt criticised for most of their lives. DBT aims to pull these extremes together so the patient learns not to hide nor overtly express feelings, to express how they feel, become less critical of others and less self-critical.

In DBT the relationship between therapist and patient is cooperative as they deal with a patient's core beliefs. DBT develops positive behaviour, promotes self-understanding and offers reward through praise. DBT builds on individual success and spreads change throughout formerly unproductive behaviour. DBT is complex therapy carried out by a team of therapists in individual or group sessions comprising 4 arms:

- learning to tolerate distress
- mindfulness – based on Buddhist 'keeping in the moment'
- the regulation of emotions
- inter-personal effectiveness

Cognitive Therapies

Cognitive therapists attribute frustrations, anxieties and emotional problems to faulty thinking patterns. These stem from dysfunctional childhoods or traumatic life experiences. Cognitive therapy is an approach which encourages patients to recognize, challenge and ultimately re-think their negative thoughts and the associated negative emotions and behaviour. Behavioural and cognitive therapies have been combined into cognitive-behavioural therapy (CBT), which used to combat stress disorders and mild to moderate depression.

21st Century – Virtual Brain Simulation

Real hope for rapid progress in the treatment of mental illness has come about through attempts to build maps of the brain using computer simulation (virtual brains). This stimulate faster research into the faulty genes responsible for serious illness like MDP or schizophrenia. Such research would normally take decades but computers vastly speed this work. Perhaps we are nearing the time when mental illness becomes a thing of the past, like polio.

DNA Research

Research into the biochemistry of the brain is bringing a sea change in the treatment of mental disorders. Scientists are using an increasing understanding of DNA to make headway into the cause and potential cures for mental illness. Drugs are more effective, side effects lessened and there is increased knowledge around the complexities involved when chemicals are combined.

Psychopathic Personality Disorder and the Law

In early 2012 there was an interesting programme about the chemistry of psychopathic personality disorder (PPD). Although this disorder lies outside the subject matter of this book the discoveries have relevance to the increasing complexity of the relationship between mental illness, ethics and the law. Two chemicals have been discovered as probable causes of PPD. This means that in the future PPD might become treatable. What comes next runs into ethics:

• how far should science interfere with personality
• how would this be achieved on moral and social grounds
• how would this affect the law

In Tennessee a man convicted of murder was found to have the psychopathic gene. The jury convicted him of manslaughter but not murder - because he lacked the conscience gene.

As the scientist involved explained, there is a great deal of difference between chemical factors and wilfulness. He expressed concerns how this might be viewed by courts and whether in the future it might literally be possible to 'get away with murder'.

Therapeutic Relationship

The positive influence of a good therapeutic relationship has been acknowledged since the talking cures came into fashion. It is scientifically recognised as a phenomenon with vital importance in healing. During Professor Kathy Sykes Channel 4 programmes CAT scans of patients showed pain centres in nerve endings reduced during spiritual healing sessions. Similar discoveries were made about acupuncture points. Spiritual healing resembles a therapeutic relationship. It is also not dissimilar to a healing method of American Indians called a 'pow wow', where members of a tribe gathered to listen sympathetically and resolve fellow tribesmen's problems.

Neuro-Typical v Non Neuro-typical

The argument about what is 'normal' (sane) is ongoing. With the discovery of conditions such as autism and high functioning autism there has been more public awareness of alternative realities.

Psychiatrists are used to putting clusters of symptoms into bands which describe illness, such as schizophrenia, but these categories have overlaps, making diagnosis difficult. New thinking borne out by research holds there is no such thing as neuro-typical; everyone has a kind of pathology. With this comes a move toward the isolation and treatment of individual symptoms, rather than an arbitrary attempt to divide mental disorders into clusters of symptoms.

A Personal Experience of Labelling

A label is a diagnostic tool and also an explanation of a quality or state. Labelling or naming a disorder is vital to enable research, understanding, treatment and cure.

I would be more anxious if I did not know my life has been so different to that of my peers, why I was ridiculed and bullied so often for 'being different' and why no one ever told me I had autism.

A label acknowledges the suffering which comes with disorders such as Aspergers and somehow validates it. Finally it enables engagement with support organisations and peers. The argument for and against labels will no doubt continue.

Chapter 5
The Mental Health Act 1983

Content:
Overview
Definitions of Staff within the Act:
Sections of the Mental Health Act

What follows is a very brief overview of the legislation underpinning the sectioning of patients in the now defunct 1983 Act. Although the Act is defunct, it is an important part of the history of mental illness. This act serves to highlight the legal and moral issues surrounding the treatment of the mentally ill in the community and raises interesting questions which are useful to those new to the field.

The Mental Health Act was brought into being to protect the public and those who might harm themselves during an episode of mental illness. Under its terms people who were considered a danger to themselves or the public could be removed and sent for treatment in a Psychiatric Hospital.

Overview
The Mental Health Act 1983 was set up by the Government to regulate conditions for the '*reception, care and treatment of mentally disordered patients, the management of their property and other related matters*'. The legislation was designed to protect the public from potentially dangerous patients, who might otherwise be discharged into the Community without supervision. As well as the legal part of the Act, a Code of Practice was drawn up for Health Authorities and Trusts upon which they could base their own patient care regime. The code contains:

* patient safety, privacy, dignity
* quality of care by Hospital staff
* aftercare of discharged patients
* restrictions on detained patients who self-discharge

The Mental Health Commission was tasked with overseeing recommendations and making unannounced visits to Hospitals to check standards of care. The Act was divided into Sections or chapters. Sectioning was often used as a slang verb describing how a person was taken into care i.e. 'being sectioned'.

Definitions of Staff within the Act:
The Act specified the responsibilities of each mental health professional when someone was to be sectioned. It defined the professionals and lay people who had a voice in the matter whether a relative or Court appointed official.

Approved Social Worker
A qualified Social Worker trained to make applications under the Mental Health Act and to commit under a Section of the Act.

Medical Referee
The Doctor (usually Psychiatrist) from the Hospital or it could be the patient's own General Practitioner. If a second reference was required this person had to be from a different Hospital and not a subordinate of the first Doctor. These measures were to:
- prevent colleagues agreeing to a Section
- prevent embarrassment if a junior disagreed with a senior

Medical Referees could not be relatives or gain financially from patients.

Mental Health Managers (MHM)
If the Hospital was run by a Trust, the MHM was the Trust Board.

Mental Health Review Tribunal (MHRT)
Tribunal consisted of professional and lay members (members of the public). Tribunals were appointed by the Lord Chancellor.

Nearest Relative
The nearest relative was a close relative of the patient who might be a partner, spouse or parent. If a spouse they had to be living with the patient for at least 6 months and be over 18 years old. If no relative existed the Courts appointed someone to act in that capacity.

Responsible Medical Officer (RMO)
The person responsible for the medical care was usually a GP.

Sections of the Mental Health Act
As you read the terms try to imagine it happening to you or a close relative. Consider the vulnerabilities of patient and relatives. Applications allowing someone to be admitted to Psychiatric Hospital

for treatment were made by an Approved Social Worker, Psychiatrist or GP who had seen the patient in the prior 14 days.

Section 2 – Admission for Assessment
Two Doctors could detain a person for 28 days under Section 2. 28 days was a long time for anyone to be held in a Psychiatric Hospital for the first time.

Could you cope with 28 days in the presence of un-medicated severely ill patients? Staff would be used to strange behaviour but to someone newly ill this could appear frightening.

Section 3 – Admission for Treatment
Section Three was admission up to six months with extensions for six months then periods of a year. This is how some detainees spent huge tracts of time in hospital. Tribunals consisted of professionals and lay people. This Section could be objected to by a patient's near relative.

Imagine waiting for a Tribunal. If the result was unfavourable your case might not be considered for a whole year. Imagine being a relative; would you have the confidence to oppose a decision made by a professional? Under what grounds would you feel this possible?

Section 4 – Emergency admission
This emergency Section required the agreement of a Medical Referee who could detain for 3 days.

What if that Doctor was overtired, did not know the patient and had to make a hurried decision? What if the patient was of a different culture or unconventional? Might this colour your perception? Remember these were life changing decisions.

Section 20 – Renewal (of a Section)
This section applied if a Doctor considered the patient might improve if they were held for 6 months or one year periods thereafter. The renewal was aimed to protect the patient and the wider public from potential harm.

Imagine someone detained for months or years. It was common for people to become institutionalized, that is, so used to living in hospital they were unable to cope in the community. Asylums protected people from cruelty but also affected a return to normal life.

Section 23 – Discharge
Discharge was lengthy and involved a Tribunal. Relatives had a say but could be overruled by the Medical Referee or Tribunal.

Consider how difficult it might be for a patient to prove they could cope. Might professionals be looking for illness rather than wellness?

Would misinterpretations be possible? Might a patient afraid to face the community have a vested interest in remaining sectioned?

Sections 57 Consent to Treatment

This Section was consent to brain surgery (or hormonal implants in the case of a sex offender). The patient had to give voluntary consent. Three Psychiatrists had to give a good case that treatment would alleviate the condition.

Consent by the patient depended upon how well the Doctor convinced them of the efficacy of treatment and an honest opinion on negative implications. But with little alternative, what could they do?

Section 58 Consent to Treatment

Section 58 was consent for medication or ECT (Electro Convulsive Therapy). Patients had to give informed consent which means they were given information about the treatment and likely risks. In cases where the patient was insufficiently mentally aware, the Mental Health Act Commission appointed a Second Opinion Doctor to act on behalf of the patient. He or she might give a go-ahead, even if the patient refused permission for this treatment.

Section 93 - 113 Financial Affairs of Sectioned Patients

In some cases, a Court of Protection appointed a professional with Power of Attorney over a patient i.e. CoP gave legal permission for someone to manage the finances of a patient. In all cases, the persons appointed had to keep financial records and report to the Court and were required to act 'in the best interests of the patient'.

Imagine you are mentally ill but you have lucid moments when you are aware of what is happening. You realize someone is looking after your finances. Would that make you feel vulnerable? Would it be easy to feel demoralised and regress, forcing a relative to care for you?

Section 134 – Withholding of Correspondence

This Section included:
- the right to open & withhold patients' outgoing mail (if the addressee said they did not wish to receive mail from a patient)
- ditto, if the MHAM felt mail would distress the addressee
- right of the Mental Health Act Managers (MHAM)to withhold incoming mail in the interests of safety

Accurate records were kept about withheld mail. Mail addressed to MPs or legal advisers had to be delivered unless they gave written instruction to the contrary. This maintained the patient's right to contact their MP or solicitor. The patient could appeal to the Mental Health Act Commission for restoration of delivery, except where the addressee had instructed otherwise.

Manic patients might send letters may with outrageous sexual content or highly personal remarks. *In these circumstances what is your opinion regarding Royal Mail's duty to accept and deliver mail despite a recipient's objection? Would you want such mail? What if a deluded patient was seeking bomb making equipment, guns or knives?*

Section 135 – Power to Enter (Private) premises
A Warrant had to be obtained by an Approved Social Worker (ASW) from a Justice of the Peace;
- police could enter premises by force if necessary
- police, approved social worker & doctor to be present
- patient was taken into a place of safety
- patient could be held for up to 72 hours (3 days)

This Section dealt with persons in private premises believed to need urgent treatment. Sections were not issued lightly, but medical opinions might vary about severity of illness.

Imagine you feel safe in your home although you are experiencing symptoms. You are taken from your home without warning.

Imagine the distress of living with someone with bizarre or even dangerous symptoms. Your relative might have attempted suicide or spent large amounts of money under the influence of a manic illness.

Families might wait a considerable time until an illness was considered serious enough to warrant Sectioning. The only other option would be to persuade their relative to go to hospital, in practice extremely difficult if the relative was psychotic.

Section 136 – Removal of People from Public Places
Police could remove someone from a public area for mental health assessment. The patient might be kept in a place of safety for up to 72 hours (3 days). This was controversial. Multi-cultural Communities had different social, spiritual and religious beliefs and there was room for misinterpretation of behaviour (remember the robed man in my example).
Police officers were not trained Mental Health workers although Health Authorities provided basic training.

In extremist regimes many have been detained for political reasons under such Acts.

How could abuse be prevented? Would you put public safety over individual freedom? How would you react if your relative was held? What would you do if your relative refused to go to hospital but was not ill enough to be sectioned?

So the Act, though set in law, was not so easy to administer and there were many moral issues and many frustrations, for patients and relatives. In the 21st century, with terrorism, migrations of different cultures into what will be alien landscapes, the question of how to deal with psychotic or suicidal patients becomes ever more difficult.

Chapter 6

From Detection to Diagnosis

Content:
How Mental Illness is Detected
Mind (*function of the brain*)
Diagnosis (Case History, Examination, DSM Manual)
Undisclosed Cases of Mental Illness

How Mental Illness is Detected

Mental illness has to be discovered before proper diagnosis can be made. Whilst this might seem obvious, in many cases those with symptoms never come forward or are treated (or hidden) within their family or community.

Two important factors which might indicate mental illness are changes in behaviour and mood. These include greater tiredness or increased energy; withdrawing from company or becoming outrageous; irritability, over excitement or lethargy. Slight differences might be normal mood changes but when these changes become marked, with no inciting events such as bereavement, marriage or birth, they may require treatment.

The most obvious people to notice changes are family, friends and close colleagues. Perhaps an employer might notice an employee whose work is deteriorating with no obvious cause. A family member might notice a relative becoming withdrawn or hyperactive. Perhaps a friend might notice changes in mood; someone outgoing becoming withdrawn or a quiet person becoming outrageous or pugnacious.

So how does detection of mental illness happen? Anyone can:

- go to their GP if they are worried about their health
- be taken by friends or family to a Psychiatric Hospital
- be detained under a Mental Health Act, if acting outrageously or dangerously in a public place

The initial diagnosis can be made by a GP or (less often) through direct referral to a Community Mental Health Team. Informally referred patients can be seen at home, in a GP Surgery or a consulting room in a Psychiatric Hospital. It is not always a Psychiatrist who diagnoses in a team setting, although [s]he is clinically responsible and will be the most qualified to prescribe medication. However, a GP retains clinical responsibility throughout treatment.

Physical and Mental Diagnoses

Diagnosis is '*the identification of disease by an investigation of symptoms and history*'. In physical illness/ disability, a General Practitioner has many clues to help diagnosis. If a patient has a painful leg and the GP sees bruising and swelling and has recently fallen whilst skiing the GP might conclude '*You have a suspected fracture*'. The patient, duly grateful, would comply by having an x-ray, possibly followed by a plaster cast, bed rest and physiotherapy. His relatives visit the hospital and be grateful at the end of treatment.   Where the symptoms are mental rather than physical things are not clear cut.

If a GP said to his patient '*I'm afraid you are mentally ill*', the patient might not believe him and resist treatment, especially if this involved being incarcerated in Psychiatric Hospital. Perhaps they would object to being thought 'mad' (colloquial). Mental Illness unfortunately still carries a stigma. Diagnosis of mental illness is difficult and takes far longer than the diagnosis of medical problems.

Mind (*function of the brain*)

The brain is a delicate instrument.   This control centre governs thoughts, feelings and actions. It also controls the autonomous nervous system (automatic systems like breathing, heartbeat, the cough reflex). The brain is in continual use from pre-birth to the moment of death, both waking and sleeping. Small wonder it occasionally malfunctions.

Mental illness affects majorly the mind. No one knows for certain where the *mind* is sited, although it is generally accepted to be within the brain. This is not as bizarre as it sounds, for some evidence has been found for nerve pathways and memory in other parts of the body.

Mind is where consciousness (awareness) occurs. The brain stem (base of the brain) contains the unconscious mind and our primitive survival mechanisms. Although much has been discovered about genetics and neurons (electrical messengers of the brain),we know very little about mental processes or how they relate to stimuli.

It is widely accepted that mental illness is a complex product of internal and external factors, including thinking, experience, environment, genes and resilience. Some of these factors can be manipulated whilst others remain outside our control.

Diagnoses take into account many factors apart from the obvious behavioural/emotional ones. Culture, profession, life experience, environment, attitudes and believes are important factors to be taken into consideration. Finally there is a vulnerability factor; if the patient had prior episodes of mental illness, if they have no supportive family or friends, lack of support in the community.

Even after diagnosis, there may be problems with treatment. Brain and mind are both as unreliable as any machine. They do not always take you safely where you want to go.

Diagnosis (Case History, Examination, DSM Manual)

Case History
The first action of a GP or Psychiatrist is to take a case history:
- the nature of the problem(s)
- how the patient believes these problems occurred
- the patient's physical and mental health
- if they have noticed changes in mood and behaviour

The diagnostician considers the medical history in order to establish:

- where the problems might have started
- how well the patient is able to deal with problems
- if there are pre existing illnesses or diseases
- how long the illness has lasted
- the level of the problem and its likely outcome

Physical Examination
A professional might make blood and psychological tests as well as a physical examination. Mental illness can co-exist with physical disorders and one can affect the other.

Medical Diagnosis

Finally the professional is ready to apply these factors and diagnose i.e. put a name to the illness.

Diagnostic & Statistics Manual [DSM]
One of the tools a Psychiatrist uses is a book called *Diagnostic and Statistics Manual* (DSM) the current being DSM IV. This American manual lists the conditions (criteria) present in all known psychiatric disorders. It is a kind of servicing manual – it lets the professional know what to look for, and includes a range of symptom severity.

Guidelines in DSM have been arrived at through research and observation. Each condition has a set of identifying numbers and letters allowing systematic diagnosis. The diagnostician will also apply clinical knowledge and life experience, as well as cultural factors and the known character traits of their patient.

DSM changes over time. Trends change with social attitudes and with new scientific discoveries. For example plans are afoot to reassess the autistic spectrum, replacing individual diagnoses with symptom clusters. Homosexuality once appeared as a diagnosis whereas most societies now class this as an accepted form of sexuality. Bulimia and Anorexia have been amalgamated under the heading of eating disorders. It is likely that personality disorders will eventually be removed from the DSM. Personality has many factors outside pathology, including culture, moral judgements and 'norms'.

Undisclosed Cases of Mental Illness

Mental illness can be only be treated when a potential patients presents to a GP or Psychiatrist. Many people who might receive treatment remain 'hidden' for a variety of reasons:

- family or friends tolerate eccentric behaviour
- symptoms pass for normal in dysfunctional families
- mild to moderate depression is viewed as normal sadness
- mania passes for exuberant or high spirits
- in certain cultures, the ill person is looked after at home
- if mental illness is seen as shameful, they might be 'hidden' at home
- mood or behaviour go unnoticed in isolated individuals
- symptoms might spontaneously disappear
- many folk with mental illness choose solitary lifestyles
  (this does not mean all solitary types have mental illness!)

There is no evidence that mental illness is only faulty genes. It is generally accepted that vulnerability stems from a combination of exterior circumstances and environmental factors. What mental illness is NOT is weakness of character. I am happy to scotch that myth.

Chapter 7
Non Medical Therapists – Talking Cures

Content:
What is a Therapist?
Psycho Analyst
Psychotherapist
Psychologist
Cognitive Behavioural Therapist
Counsellor
Empathy
Mental Health Rehabilitation Worker
Social Worker

Severe or chronic symptoms like psychoses and delusions are treated with medication (which act at chemical level). Psychiatric drugs were not available until the 1950's. Prior to that, mental illness was treated with talking cures or isolation. Post 20th century, medication is used only for serious symptoms, the rest being treated with talking therapies or complementary therapies. Most patients prefer treatment in the community or at a GP surgery, because of the stigma surrounding hospitalization or psychiatric hospitals.

What is a Therapist?
A therapy, according to my Oxford Illustrated Dictionary, is 'a If a patient is referred to a Community Mental Health Team a Therapist is chosen for them. The Team meets weekly to discuss new cases and decide who is suitable and has space. Those who pay privately can choose a Therapist.

Length of training
Length of training varies but:
- younger therapists have less life experience
- the relationship between client and Therapist is vital

Is Personal Experience – Vital for therapists?
Imagine taking a Ford car to a mechanic. His theory is sound, he has repaired many cars during training. He will repair it adequately because a Ford is a popular car and well known by most mechanics. Now imagine your car is a Porsche and your mechanic races cars and

has re-built his own engine and also has a certificate from the maker. In other words he has specialist knowledge. Considering the value of your car to whom would you entrust the repairs, a standard mechanic or a specialist?

The brain is like a finely tuned engine. When it ceases to function we call that phenomenon, mental illness. There are a wide range of mental illnesses some more serious than others. Some come and go (episodic) whilst others are lifelong (chronic) and incurable. There are social symptoms and behavioural symptoms as well as physical symptoms. This is what makes diagnosis difficult and why it should be undertaken only by a competent person. As an aside, I've met competent persons who are unqualified medically and incompetent persons who are qualified, so even that is difficult to determine.

Empathy

When selecting a Therapist, there are two vital criteria. Therapists who have unresolved life problems will not help anyone. Therapists with wide life experience are more likely to have a quality called empathy; good therapists possess this in spades. Empathy is not sympathy but an ability to understand someone's suffering without being emotionally crushed or remaining detached. The best talking therapist is always someone the patient instinctively respects.

Psycho Analyst

Psycho Analysts (followers of Sigmund Freud) are very rarely available on the NHS. The training is extensive and expensive. An Analyst undergoes a training analysis lasting several years and fully training an Analyst is reckoned to take about 10 years.

Psycho = of the mind; analysis = investigation.

Analysts investigate a sick (neurotic) mind by analysing mental processes. An Analyst's job is to help patients become aware of the unconscious mental processes which lead to problems. As mental processes cannot be observed, an Analyst investigates them via:

- **emotions** - emotions expressed when talking about difficult subjects
            e.g. they become angry when talking about parents
- **thoughts** - patients free associate - revealing problematic areas
- **fantasies and dreams** –dreams reveal hidden facts or situations

Psychotherapist

All schools of psychotherapy stem from Freud and Jung. It is impossible to generalise in a few lines but there are many primer books on the subject.

Psychotherapy is a talking cure. The patient/client speaks, writes, acts or otherwise communicates his difficulties to the Therapist. Some Psychotherapists use an Integrative method, that is, one which is based on more than one school of thought. The work of the therapist is to help the patient understand why their problems occur. With benefit of insight (understanding) the patient learns to recognise and change negative situations and put this into practice in daily life. This is not a short therapy and might take months or even years.

Psychotherapy patients might go for therapy to deal with a specific difficulty, whereas Analysands (psycho analytic patients) spend years in analysis to gain deep insight and understand themselves fully.

Psychotherapy involves talking about difficult and emotional situations. Length of therapy depends on the nature of the problem and how hard the patient works at it. Psychotherapy is sometimes available on the NHS through a GP application for special funding.

Psychologist

Psychology is the study of human behaviour and is rooted in Jung's work. Psychologists appear in different areas; education, employment, forensic (criminal) work, mental health. Psychologists study animal behaviour and apply this knowledge to humans. They are interested in behaviour, environment and family.

Cognitive Behavioural Therapist

Cognitive behavioural therapy involves a patient learning to recognize their faulty thinking patterns and changing behaviour that led to the problem. CBT puts faulty thinking and behaviour at the root of human discontent. Clinical Psychologists work in hospitals. They study for three to four year for an Honours Degree in Psychology and can then specialise, for example taking further training as a Registered Clinical Psychologist to work with hospital patients.

Psychologists work in research and publish professional papers on mental health issues. All Clinical Psychologists in the UK have to be registered.

Counsellor

The roots of Counselling lie in the village wise women of earlier times. The seeker consulted a wise woman and received common sense advice based on tribal culture and would be offered charms or herbs. Although counselling began as a complementary therapy Counsellors are commonly found in the NHS, University, GP Surgeries and private hospitals. Counselling as a talking cure stemmed from the work of Breur, Jung and Freud.

Counselling takes many forms according to training and convention. It is based on the *therapeutic relationship* between client and therapist. Some forms are brief, based on the work of Milton Erickson. Others are of longer duration, based on the principles of Freud and Jung. The type of counselling appropriate depends upon the type of problem being presented, its severity and duration. These factors are decided by the practitioner to whom the patient is presented in the NHS, or by choice in the private sector.

Counselling is an effective treatment for mild to moderate depression, emotional difficulties, bereavement, traumas connected with natural disasters or practical concerns. Other patients are the so called *worried well* with stress or anxieties and not full blown mental illness. Counselling is not used in treating psychosis, depression of suicidal level or obsessions which respond better to medication.

Empathy

Those who have a great deal of life experience make the best talking therapists. Therapists who have problems and do not realize it or do nothing about it are not helping anyone, because they have blind spots. The best way of selecting a talking therapist is someone the patient respects. When considering therapists for the talking therapies you need to consider - has that person a deep understanding of the problem. Empathy is not the same as sympathy. Empathy is an ability to understand someone's suffering without being emotionally crushed by that experience.

Mental Health Rehabilitation Worker

Rehabilitation Workers (Rehabs.) used to receive on the job training on unqualified Social Workers scales but there is now a City and Guilds Qualification in mental rehabilitation. They are chosen for their maturity and breadth of life experience.

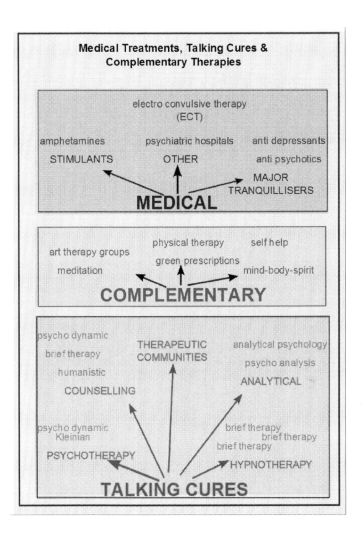

Rehabs in the UK work within a Mental Health Team and gather cases which do not readily fall into the other disciplines. Mostly, their caseload consists of patients with long-term mental illness who need Social Skills Training but they also take on short-term outpatients. A rehab's job might be considered as one of social education and social support.

Social Worker

Social Work trainees have to be 22 years of age with some experience of working in the field or voluntary work. A degree in Social Work takes three years; the trainee gains a Degree (DipSW) in Social Work. Their training is in social policy, welfare and legal aspects of mental health with optional training in subjects such as addictions, psychology or learning disability. Social Worker trainees have to spend a proportion of their training on-the-job. Social Workers help patients with problems of day-to-day living. They might deal with housing, benefits, neighbour disputes, and general behavioural problems. Although there is a mild tag of social work being work done with working people they in fact work across the spectrum, also working with outpatients who do not have chronic mental health conditions. Social Workers make legal applications for Sectioning under the Mental Health Act.

Chapter 8
Medical Practitioners

Content:
Psychiatrist
General Practitioner
Registered Mental Nurse
Pharmacist

Medically qualified practitioners are the only professionals who can legally prescribe psychiatric drugs, though this may vary according to training. A special drugs training is required for other practitioners to prescribe. The work of non medical mental health professionals was described in the previous chapter. The next chapter covers treatments offered by the medical profession.

Psychiatrist

A Psychiatrist trains in General Medicine and obtains a Doctorate. After qualifying they spend a year in General Practice before taking the extra training to enable them to become Junior Psychiatrists (6 months). It then takes around 5 years to become a Consultant. Psychiatrists are trained in all aspects of brain chemistry and the drugs used to treat mental illness. They train in analytical or psychological therapies and underpinning cultural knowledge and laws. Some go on to train in brain surgery or specialize in organic brain disorders such as Alzheimer's or forensic (criminal) psychiatry. A Psychiatrist administers ECT (electro convulsive therapy).

Some senior Mental Nurses take training in psychiatric medication. Psychiatric medication is powerful and dangerous in the wrong hands but sadly this does not seem to deter people selling it or buying it, often at huge risk.

General Practitioner

General Practitioner training lasts about seven years comprising examinations and on-the-job training in hospitals). Competition for Medical School is high and entrants have to achieve good science grades for MBBS Doctorate training. General Practitioners study anatomy, physiology and biology as well as a specialist subject.

Psychiatrists are qualified Doctors who have taken extra training in psychiatric medicine. Doctor refers to the Degree or Doctorate in Medicine (MD). The term Doctor is used colloquially – i.e. '*I went to my Doctor the other day*' but this is incorrect use of the term.

Registered Mental Nurse

Registered Mental Nurses have a 3 year training partly classroom based and partly in the field. They are taught to recognise symptoms of major mental illnesses and treatments such as behavioural therapies. At present it is more usual for a GP or Psychiatrist to prescribe but Advanced Practitioners are now allowed to do so. Mental Nurses diagnose under Supervision from a Consultant Psychiatrist. They work in a Community Mental Health Team (CMHT) attached to a local Psychiatric Hospital. Incidentally do you know how trainee nurses practice giving injections? They inject oranges until deemed fit to practice on patients.

Pharmacist

Pharmacists are scientists who specialise in the preparation and dispensing of medicines (drugs). Their profession dates back to the early Nineteenth Century when practitioners were variously known as Apothecaries or Druggists or Chemists. Pharmacists work in Research Laboratories, Hospitals or Community Pharmacies. The latter is either a specialist shop, part of a Chemist's Shop or maybe a supermarket. Students with excellent passes in science subjects such as chemistry and physics take a four year Master of Pharmacy Honours Degree (plus one year post degree training.

- physical properties of chemicals
- chemistry of pharmaceuticals (drugs used as medicines)
- reaction of these chemicals in the human body
- how to measure correct doses

Pharmacists can now prescribe certain medications if they have suitable training but this does not include restricted drugs such as cocaine and heroin. They can only prescribe within their medical competence, which does not include psychiatric medication unless they have the necessary training. However, they can override a GP's prescription for drugs, where the Pharmacist has reason to believe the GP has prescribed wrongly or has proposed a drug incompatible with medication the patient is currently taking (contra indication).

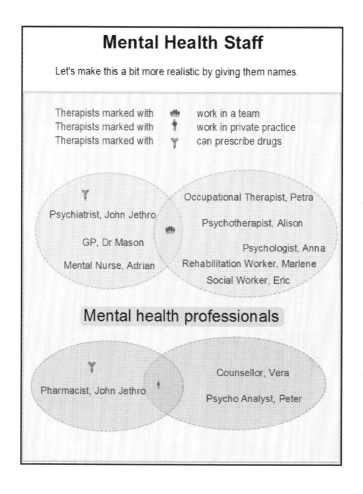

Mental Health Staff

Let's make this a bit more realistic by giving them names.

Therapists marked with 🏶 work in a team
Therapists marked with 👤 work in private practice
Therapists marked with ⚕ can prescribe drugs

⚕
Psychiatrist, John Jethro
GP, Dr Mason
Mental Nurse, Adrian

Occupational Therapist, Petra
Psychotherapist, Alison
Psychologist, Anna
Rehabilitation Worker, Marlene
Social Worker, Eric

🏶

Mental health professionals

⚕
Pharmacist, John Jethro

Counsellor, Vera
Psycho Analyst, Peter

Chapter 9
Modern Medical Treatments

Content:
Brain Chemistry Imbalance
Electro Convulsive Therapy (ECT)
Modern Drug Therapies
Designing New Drugs
Stages of a Drug Trial
Categories of Drugs for Sale
Drug Groups
Psychosurgery
Medical Practitioners

Medicine has largely taken over the treatment of enduring mental illness. But even medications change as old ones fall out of favour in the light of new discoveries, not least the genetic code, neurology and more in-depth knowledge of how the mind works. Modern medical treatments include:

- psychology/ psychotherapy/ counselling (the 'talking cures')
- drug therapies (medication - pharmaceuticals)
- psychosurgery (brain surgery)
- electro convulsive therapy (ECT)

Brain Chemistry Imbalance
It is known among mental health professionals that brain chemistry affects mood and behaviour. But mood and behaviour changes are normal functions. Humans are vital beings who respond to the environment. Unable to adapt, we would have no opinions, no will or ability to adapt to a changing environment, still less garner an appreciation of subjective experiences like art, beauty and love. Mood and behaviour changes enable us to adapt, show appreciation and move forward from our raw animal heritage. Repetitive change allows us to explore, invent, experiment, philosophise and overcome life circumstances and not least to live harmoniously in communities.

However, extreme imbalances in brain chemistry can wreak havoc. Sometimes people become so overwhelmed with inner turmoil they are unable to function properly, causing difficulties for themselves and others. In a few cases, they might become a danger to themselves or society. Only extreme states are classed as enduring mental illness. The effects of normal life traumas such as bereavement or the end of a relationship are passing states generally even out. Traumatic events, sometimes referred to as life events, are part of being human but sometimes the shock triggers an underlying condition. This is not a cause for concern, because the condition can then be treated. As a case in point, I cite my own diagnosis of autism. Look at the diagram following on brain chemistry imbalance. This explains how brain chemistry can alter for many reasons. Diet, drugs and alcohol are also known to affect brain chemistry (think diabetes, for instance). There are other contributory factors:

- birthing problems
- faulty genes
- accidental injury to the brain
- poverty, poor housing, severe life stress

There is NO evidence that social standing or education have a bearing on mental illness. If social standing were the case, none of the Royal Family would have been diagnosed with mental illness! However, the traumatic effects of extreme poverty and poor environments ARE linked to incidents of mental illness. You might be aware of an old misnomer which states 'poor people are mad, the rich merely eccentric'. Mental illness has no boundaries.

Even medical practitioners are coming round to something long understood by holistic practitioners, that all three elements of mind, body and spirit need attention, as problems in one area have effects on the others. Holistic practitioners have long believed that the mind and body are linked and illness or imbalance in one affects the health of the other areas. 21st century therapists would generally accept this.

Electro Convulsive Therapy (ECT)

During the Roman period, patients were treated with shock therapy using electric eels. This bizarre treatment was also used in Bethlem Hospital. After the discovery of electricity by Franklin (and Edison) Psychiatrists began to experiment, hoping to shock the brains of very ill patients out of imbalance. Electrodes were attached on either side of the skull and then low electric currents were pulsed through the brain. This *electro convulsive therapy* or ECT was used with varying success for treating shell-shocked soldiers and depressive illness.

Brain Chemistry Imbalance

Brain chemistry is affected by:

1. physical environment
2. life events
3. family pathology

quality of housing

neighbours   society

continuity   nature

PHYSICAL   safety

stability **ENVIRONMENT**

workplace

OR a combination   support

of all three influences   success

dynamics   failures

attitudes

accepted behaviours   work life   disasters

FAMILY   **LIFE EVENTS**

PATHOLOGY   perceived status

emotions   upbringing   poverty

relationships

family inter-relationship   losses & bereavment

faulty genes

It was also used, up to the 1970's, to treat chronic depression which was not responding to drugs.

Normal Functioning of Chemical Transmitters
There are billions of individual cells in the brain. These are linked not physically but through the action of chemical transmitters. These chemicals form an electric current, which is seen as a wavy line on electro-encephalograph machine (EEG) readouts.

As long as each brain cell receives the right amount of chemical, it allows normal brain function. However, if for any reason, the chemical transmitters fail, it produces strong mood changes and/or bizarre behaviour, also lack of body coordination. The chemistry usually re-balances after treatment with medication or other psychiatric intervention. So brain chemistry imbalances are reversible given treatment, the equivalent of repairing wires in an electric cable.

Delivery of ECT
Early experiments with ECT looked alarming. Archive recordings showing patients convulsing as nurses hold or strap them to a table to prevent injury. Watch the movie 'A Beautiful Mind' which has a sequence of an early form of ECT being administered.

In modern ECT, a patient is given a general anaesthetic and a muscle relaxant to prevent physical injury. The currents administered are very low. Electrodes (wires attached to pads) are placed either side of the skull then connected to an ECT box which delivers the current. As the Psychiatrist switches on the current, the shock causes convulsions in the patient's muscles – it resembles an epileptic fit. A course of twelve treatments was considered beneficial.

Last Resort Treatment
From the 1950's to 1960's, ECT was regularly used to relieve the symptoms of chronic depressive illness and schizophrenia. At this time there were few drugs and the only other treatment was incarceration in an Asylum. No one knew how ECT worked, only that it did in a small number of cases. Even then it was controversial, because of the serious side effects of memory loss and personality change. 1950's wards were filled with patients damaged through excessive use of ECT. Once drug therapy was introduced, ECT was discontinued except for extreme cases. Where it is used, modern ECT delivers a current on one side of the brain, at low voltage.

The Human Brain: 1

There are billions of synapes or connections in the brain, depicted in the schematic diagram below. Each is capable of growing an infinite number of the hair-like structures which carry signals to the brain. These signals or electrical pulses can be seen on an EEG machine readout.

Signals are triggered by thoughts, autonomic reactions like breathing, or muscular impulses from various parts of the body.

each synapse is not physically connected. Chemical transmitters 'fire' across the gaps like an electric current, carrying 'messages' which react to a specific need, whether triggered by a thought or an automatic body function.

Modern Drug Therapies
What are Drugs?
Drugs are chemicals designed by scientist-chemists in pharmaceutical companies to treat specific illnesses. Drugs for mental illnesses work by interacting at neuro-transmitter level on brain chemistry. New drugs have to be tested for years, sometimes over a decade, and must pass stringent tests before they are allowed onto the market. The slang term *drug* is sometimes used when describing illegal use of medication. Morphine, heroin, cocaine are legal drugs used by medical professionals for the relief of pain. When they get into the wrong hands for recreational use, they become illegal.

All drugs have curative and harmful properties. The harmful properties are referred to as side effects. Sometimes the medical profession make errors and prescribe wrong doses or a fail to take account of a medication which reacts adversely to another drug or even a particular food (contra-indication). All drugs have side effects because combining chemicals changes their properties, sometimes in ways unexpected even by the scientists.

Psychiatric drugs replace depleted mood-changing chemicals. When delivered in the right quantities over a longish period, the brain generally recovers. When brain chemistry recovers, drugs can be withdrawn, however if drugs are withdrawn too quickly there will be a relapse. It takes months to allow the brain transmitters to begin working properly This is why it is vital for patients to adhere to instructions and not stop taking medication until advised by a professional.

Designing New Drugs
New drugs appear regularly. Anyone using a brand for a long time will notice how from time to time their GP prescribes a new one. The pharmaceutical industry strives to improve quality and effectiveness of products, reducing side effects and testing new molecules for beneficial properties. There are huge costs involved in the design of new drugs, many of which never come onto the market, for reasons of safety or marketability. Drugs which prove interesting in the laboratory might fail human trials and are withdrawn. Refer to the diagrams following, which show the progress of a new drug trial.

The Human Brain: 2

If the chemical transmitter, for various reasons, fails to 'jump' the gap between synapses, that part of the brain ceases to function as it should.

For example:
* mood might be affected
* a limb may fail to move when directed by a thought
* a memory might be blocked
* an organ might malfunction

Mood changes can be caused by faulty or too low concentrations of mood-enhancing chemical transmitters. These are referred to by Doctors as an 'imbalance of brain chemistry'. Anti depressant and other drugs are designed to redress these imbalances.

Stages of a Drug Trial
Preliminary– discovery and animal testing

Every Pharmaceutical Company has laboratories where scientists create new drug molecules. Molecules are the small particles from which all matter (material) is made. If a chemical looks promising scientists first develop a new drug then conduct animal tests to see if benefits outweigh negative effects. Initial testing is carried out on laboratory rats, mice or dogs. A few companies only test on humans but this is only on drugs containing proven chemicals.

Scientists are looking for signs of toxicity (harmful) and mutagenicity (whether it alters or mutates the structure of the organism). Careful documentation is kept at every stage and these are scrutinized by drug licensing authorities. Even the smallest error on applications can lead to rejection of the whole drug trial, for the sake of safety.

Phase 1 Testing – on volunteers

After the preliminary stage, stage 1 tests are carried out on healthy humans. Sometimes these are volunteers among the pharmaceutical company's employees. They must remain on laboratory premises for the duration of testing. Outside volunteers are paid well for taking part in trials. Very toxic drugs such as those designed for treating cancer are tested only on patients (i.e. people who have the disease).

Volunteer trials are aimed at discovering:

- how toxic the drug is, i.e. how well the body tolerates it
- how the body disposes of the drug
- comparative responses with people given blind trials *

blind (placebo) - harmless substances are given certain volunteers to compare their response that of volunteers actually given the drug.

- how the body disposes of the drug
- comparative responses with people given blind trials *

blind or placebo tests where harmless substances are given certain volunteers to compare their response that of volunteers actually given the drug.

A drug trial was halted a few years ago when volunteer patients developed pain within minutes of the drug being administered. The drug had been tested but something went wrong.

Under such circumstances the trial is halted and an investigation takes place. Sometimes a drug is taken to a certain stage but a rival company gets to market first. When Viagra took the market by storm, a rival laboratory quietly stopped trials for its own product, Erecnos. May be just as well, considering the excruciating name.

Phase 2 Testing – on patients

Once volunteer trials have concluded phase 2 tests commence on a small number of patients who have the relevant disease and have given consent to take part. If trials are successful, more patients are recruited. Applications are made for permission to make alternations to the procedure as trials progress.

Tests on patients show if drugs are effective, dosages at which they work and negative effects. Every drug has negative effects as currently it is impossible to *synthesize* (combine) chemicals and only have positive benefits. If a drug has more side effects than positive ones, the trials will be ended.

Phase 3 – large scale testing on human patients

This is an important part of the drug trial procedure and determines whether the new drug is allowed a license, without which it cannot be sold. A large number of GP patients are asked for consent to take part in trials and are monitored for reactions to the drug. The purpose is to demonstrate if the new drug is more effective or less risky than drugs already on the market. International trials may be conducted, to gather a wide range of data. Once testing has been concluded satisfactorily a license is granted to market the drug commercially.

Phase 4 – testing after the granting of a license

Even when a license has been granted testing is not complete. The Company conducts Phase 4 tests which show up difficulties in long term use of the drug such as:

- adverse reactions in long term use
- negative effects when other drugs are used at the same time (contra indication)
- revised dosage or administration of the drug
- looking at cases where it is not effective and establishing why

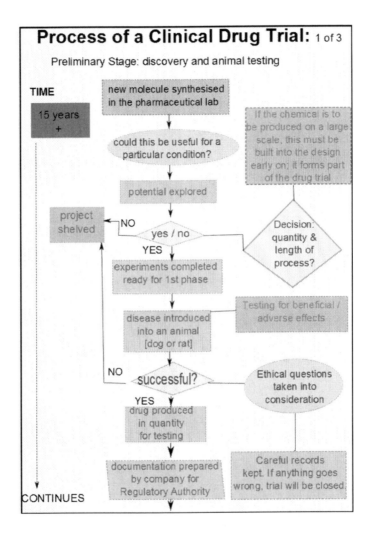

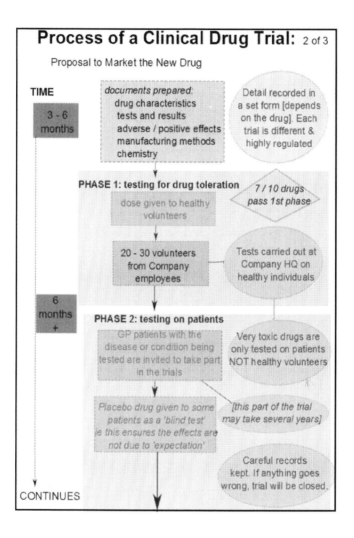

Process of a Clinical Drug Trial: 2 of 3

Proposal to Market the New Drug

TIME

3 - 6 months

documents prepared:
drug characteristics
tests and results
adverse / positive effects
manufacturing methods
chemistry

Detail recorded in a set form [depends on the drug]. Each trial is different & highly regulated

PHASE 1: testing for drug toleration

dose given to healthy volunteers

7 / 10 drugs pass 1st phase

20 - 30 volunteers from Company employees

Tests carried out at Company HQ on healthy individuals

6 months +

PHASE 2: testing on patients

GP patients with the disease or condition being tested are invited to take part in the trials

Very toxic drugs are only tested on patients NOT healthy volunteers

Placebo drug given to some patients as a 'blind test' ie this ensures the effects are not due to 'expectation'

[this part of the trial may take several years]

Careful records kept. If anything goes wrong, trial will be closed.

CONTINUES

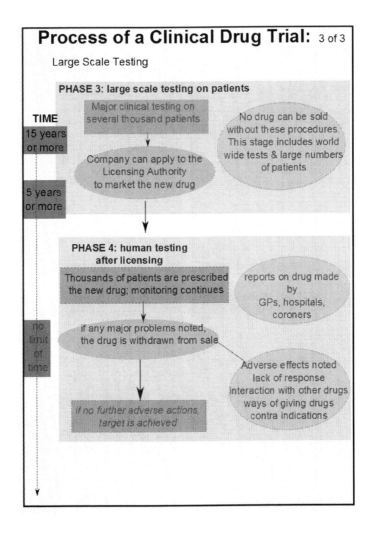

Process of a Clinical Drug Trial: 3 of 3

Large Scale Testing

PHASE 3: large scale testing on patients

TIME

15 years or more

Major clinical testing on several thousand patients

No drug can be sold without these procedures. This stage includes world wide tests & large numbers of patients

Company can apply to the Licensing Authority to market the new drug

5 years or more

PHASE 4: human testing after licensing

Thousands of patients are prescribed the new drug; monitoring continues

reports on drug made by GPs, hospitals, coroners

if any major problems noted, the drug is withdrawn from sale

no limit of time

Adverse effects noted lack of response interaction with other drugs ways of giving drugs contra indications

if no further adverse actions, target is achieved

Once large scale trials are concluded, all the negative effects are listed in MIMs (a manual used by GP's, which lists all current drugs on the market.

drugs on the market) as side effects. Even if they occur in only a few patients, all side effects must be listed by law. Side effects include headache, nausea, stomach pains, vomiting or palpitations. When a GP prescribes, they must take into account the negative effects of the drug.

Animal Testing

There has been much controversy about animal testing. In some cases drugs companies are able to conduct testing on tissue culture and thus avoid some animal research but these drugs still have to be human tested. It is questionable whether animal testing can be entirely avoided. Perhaps we had rather ask if we want to cure virulent and painful human disease/illness and knowing that animals will suffer during laboratory trials, though they try to minimalise this.

Virtual trials

I came across an article about software used by Glaxo Wellcome (one of the largest UK pharmaceuticals) which can be manipulated to simulate behaviour of individual molecules. This shortens the early stages of the drug trial. Whether it will have an impact on animal testing I am unaware and Glaxo were unable to provide an answer.

Categories of Drugs for Sale

You may wonder why certain medicines are 'prescription only' and cannot be dispensed unless in the presence of a qualified chemist. The Medicines Act 1968 lays guidelines for four classes of medicines which can be sold over the counter in the UK:

- GSL general sale list - drugs which have been used safely several years
- POM or prescription only - only on GP's prescription
- P or Pharmacy - only if the pharmacist is present
- CDPOM - dangerous drugs by GP hand written prescription

Drug Groups

The diagram on the next page shows drugs that act upon the nervous system itself. There is a selection of plants used in holistic therapies which are reputed to alleviate symptoms.

Plants, roots, bark and berries were used as medicines thousands of years before pharmaceutical drugs. Some drugs are still made from plant material.

The following are examples of botanical plants which have been used to extract pharmaceutical drugs:

- amaryllis belladonna (Belladonna Lily) –relief of Alzheimer's
- asarum canadense (wild ginger) – head colds
- curare –poisonous herb, muscle relaxant in surgery
- belladonna (deadly nightshade) –dilate pupils in eye surgery
- digitalis (foxglove) – used to regulate heart beats
- envallaria majatis (lily of the valley) – antispasmodic & diuretic
- mentha spicata (spearmint) –calming nervous disorders
- myrrhis odorata (sweet cicely) –anti cancer research trial
- salix purpurea (purple osier) –origin of aspirin
- tanacetum parthenium (feverfew) – migraine relief
- valeriana officinalis (valerian) – sedative

Wandering through the Botanic Gardens at Oxford I was struck by the beauty of these plants. Thousands of years use enabled herbalists to pass on plant therapies used to this day. This brings you in touch with man's lost relationship with nature. Three groups of drugs which act on the nervous system are:

- sedatives – suppress the nervous system
- analgesics –act as pain killers
- stimulants – stimulate the nervous system

Sedatives are commonly used in psychiatry. There are two types, anti-depressants and anti-psychotics. Anti-depressants counteract depressive illness (mood control, relief of emotional pain, promoting sleep) whilst anti-psychotics reduce hallucinations and delusions.

Antidepressants
Antidepressants relieve depressive illness but do not cure it. Depressive illness is complex and needs input such as psychological therapy and self-help. There are several kinds of anti- depressant medication which all work in different ways on the nervous system.

82

Drug Categories - drugs & herbs

barbiturates / beta blockers
diminish anxiety and reduce
paranoia

SEDATIVES

Valium   Diazapam
      Librium

Secobarbital VALERIAN

CHAMOMILE

---

major tranquillisers
treat hallucinations /
delusions

ANTI PSYCHOTICS

Largactil   Clozaril

Melleril   Serdolect

---

tranquillisers to improve mood
and relieve emotional pain

ANTI DEPRESSANTS

Seroxat   Gamanlil

Prozac   SAGE

MEADOWSWEET

---

decrease physical pain

ANALGESICS

Distalgesic   Tylenol

                     Aspirin

COMFREY

          MARIGOLD

---

stimulate nervous system
increase wakefulness

STIMULANTS

FENNEL   amphetamines

CINNAMON
          COFFEE

ALWAYS consult a Doctor
before taking any remedy,
including herbs.

KEY

DRUG CATEGORY
brand of drug within category
FOLK OR HERB REMEDY

Tricyclics
Examples of tricyclic anti depressants: Tryptizol, Sinequan.

Brain cells are connected only through chemical transmitters. This action maintains mood and behaviour. Two transmitters are serotonin and noradrenaline.

Tricyclic antidepressants increase the amount of chemical transmitter. This is like putting voltage across an electrical circuit; the appliance will power up and do its work, whether heating water or powering a drill. In the brain, chemicals enhance or repress mood, reduce unwanted behaviour and assist sleep. Tricyclic refers to the chemical structure of the drug which has a ring-like structure.

SSRI's (Specific Serotonin Re-Uptake Inhibitors)
Examples of SSRI's: Prozac, Cipramil, Seroxat.
Serotonin enhances mood.

MAOI's (monoamine oxidase inhibitors)
Example of an MAOI: Manerix, Nardil, Parnate

Monamine chemicals control the fluctuation of mood. MAO inhibitors prevent a buildup of monamines and stabilise mood.

Patient Compliance
Patients can be prescribed drugs but unless detained under a Mental Health Act, no one can be forced to take them. When patients say medication has not worked they may have broken off treatment too soon, before the chemicals have taken effect. This is common with patients taking medication for depressive illness. Even with medication, it can be months before enough chemicals are produced in the brain to enable mood to improve. If patients stop medication without professional advice, symptoms will return.

Some patients refuse medication for chronic conditions because of the side effects. These can be wide ranging and include tics, stereotypical mouth hand or body movement, heaviness or numbness, reduced sensitivity or a general inability to think clearly. You can perhaps understand why patients often do not comply. But for some patients medication is vital and without it they will not function.

In worst case scenario such as untreated schizophrenia, patients can become dangerous to themselves or others. For others, not taking medication during depressive illness prolongs their misery.

Psychosurgery

Brain operations are only carried out on very ill patients and when there is no other option. Brain operations are extremely difficult, risky and dangerous. Even in the 21st century we know relatively little about the functioning brain. However, modern psychosurgery is aided by better research into the brain, the availability of more accurate scanning equipment and very delicate instruments, including micro cameras. There are relatively few brain surgeons and operations are very expensive. Modern psychosurgery is accurate and aided by a deeper knowledge of the physical brain, accurate scanning equipment and delicate instruments including tiny cameras. Against this, there are relatively few brain surgeons and operations are very expensive to conduct.

Chapter 10
Pen Portraits of Therapists

Content of this chapter:

Vera – Private Counsellor   Anna - Clinical Psychologist
Dr Mason – G .P.   Alison - Psychotherapist
Adrian - Mental Nurse   Marlene – Rehabilitation Worker
John Jethro - Pharmacist   Eric – Social Worker
Paul Lacey – Psychiatrist   Jason – Hypno-Psychotherapist
Peter – Psycho Analyst

The following portrayals demonstrate training, practices, theory and working environment of mental health professionals in private practice and the NHS. These are fictional vignettes and not real persons, and have been simplified to demonstrate particular points. In practice, things are not so clear cut. I hope this enlivens what might otherwise be a dry section.

The first paragraph under each heading describes the training and work of the Therapist, and a fictionalised 'day in the life' follows.

Vera, Private Practice Counsellor

Vera is a Counsellor specialising in Brief Therapy. She works in private practice but also receives referrals from GP's. Her time is divided between counselling, training and running her business. She visits a Supervisor twice a week. A Supervisor provides a clinical overview of clients as well as checking Vera's mental welfare.

Brief therapists agree a fixed number of sessions with their clients, usually 1 to 8. Each lasts from 45 minutes to an hour. In some cases, clients are seen longer term but that is not strictly the brief therapy method; most Counsellors will have trained in more than one method.

Counsellors in private practice need to perform the full range of business tasks including advertising, promotion, office administration, accounts, case notes, fee-chasing, as well as attending professional training and meetings. This means very long hours. Unlike NHS staff, private practitioners do not receive a salary and pay for expenses such as Supervision, rooms, training and memberships.

*

Vera arrives at her rooms. Her client does not turn up so Vera waits in case he is late. 30 minutes later he arrives apologetically having forgotten the appointment. Vera might allow extra time, unless she judges the lateness to be a way of psychologically 'demanding more' , but more practically if no other client is due.

Tom is unhappily married and wants to talk about separating from his wife. He and his wife get on reasonably well as friends but are no longer lovers and have arguments. Tom has a 9 year old daughter and is anxious about the effect of the bad relationship on her. This session will help Tom clarify his thoughts.

By the end of the Session Tom decides on a separation and books a further session to help him work out how to provide for his family, emotionally and financially.

Vera's second client Jean is anxious about the disappearance of her daughter. Vera does not interrupt Jean's nonstop verbal stream. Jean is less anxious when she leaves having used what is a rare opportunity of airing what she feels. Over the next few days she can consider what she has said and learn more about herself in the process. Brief therapy is more directive than classic counselling but the therapist needs to know when to remain silent.

Vera's third client, Mary, has major career decisions. At the moment Mary feels overwhelmed with her children's problems which are draining her, leaving no time for her own plans. She wants a career but cannot find time to even think about this. This client is not emotionally distressed but needs practical guidance. Vera teaches Mary a problem solving techniques which she can use not only for the immediate crisis but a useful tool for the future.

After a break Vera visits a hostile Practice Manager to talk about filled rubbish bins regularly left inside the counselling room. Mrs Simmons has unpleasant ways of showing her suppressed anger to staff but has to be approached carefully or she flies into a mood. This sort of passive aggressive-behaviour to private practitioners used to be commonplace in the NHS but with more integration between the services is improving.

Vera sighs as she sees her accounts and a pile of Case Notes. Time for a break and a glance at the newspaper. She is making coffee when the phone rings. It is a GP she knows well. He is worried about a patient and wants Vera to attend as soon as possible. Vera manages to find a free spot but it means working late to catch up.

Her next call is from Tom's wife, Megan. Tom told his wife he was seeing Vera, and Megan is very angry. She wants to see Vera to talk about her husband. Vera tells her this is unethical but suggests she asks Tom if he will agree to a joint session. Megan, still angry, is insistent. Vera has to patiently explain she cannot grant this request. Megan slams down the receiver. Vera sighs. She understands Megan's frustration but is sure Tom will give permission. Megan's hoped-for reconciliation won't take place. Tom has already made his decision.

Relaxation is important for Therapists. Vera likes to watch old movies; Hammer horror and science fiction. She hasn't counselled an alien but who knows.. Vera will not spend all her career counselling. Private practice is stressful and running costs are expensive. She might teach or write or perhaps something else entirely new.

Dr Mason, General Practitioner

Dr Mason is a General Practitioner (GP) in his late 40's. He is the Senior Partner. He is qualified to diagnose, prescribe drugs and perform minor surgery. He cannot perform major surgical operations nor prescribe psychiatric drugs unless he takes additional training. Some GP's undertake training in counselling techniques or psychiatry.

Dr Mason refers patients to other specialists and acts as a clearing house between patient and specialist. He retains clinical responsibility for all his patients, which means in law he is responsible for their physical well-being. A specialist to whom Dr Mason refers a patient must report progress.

*

Dr Mason's morning Surgery starts at 8.30 am but he arrives early to clear administrative work and write notes. There are many statutory NHS forms and procedures which need attention. As each patient arrives the Receptionist finds their digitised notes. It is a legal requirement for all visits, medications and patient notes to be recorded. Dr Mason knows patients have a right to see their notes so is careful not to write anything which could be misinterpreted. Some surgeries keep separate notes for information which might prove detrimental if a patient saw them.

The Surgery is so busy. Dr Mason has 10 minutes per patient to interview, diagnosis and prescribe. Dr Mason has to be adept at interviewing. Two appointments are kept free at the end of each session for urgent appointments. When his last patient leaves Dr Mason signs repeat prescriptions, NHS forms and supervises trainees.

He might make time to see Pharmaceutical Representatives, who will be recruiting for new drug trials and want to sell new medications. A GP can prescribe new drugs so long as they are listed in MIMS (the GP's drugs manual). When Dr Mason agrees to be involved in new drug trials, he has to keep detailed records of patients who have agree to take part. The records include any positive or negative effects of the drug and whether the patient found it beneficial. This information is collated and if the drug comes onto the market, it will appear on the packaged medication under 'warnings' and in MIMS.

Dr Mason oversees Junior Doctors as part of their training. He might employ a Practice Manager to look after administration and a Fund Manager to deal with accounts and financial matters. Once a week he holds a staff meeting to discuss clinical matters. Dr Mason covers emergency callouts twice a month. Like Vera he attends a professional organization and ongoing training. Dr Mason suffers stress but unlike colleagues he has counselling when he realizes things are not right. Many GP's suffer from depression because of the working conditions – and perhaps because the medical profession attracts sensitive people with a tendency to this disorder.

Dr Mason finds it difficult to unwind. He enjoys classical music concerts and the odd game of golf. He is married with children but because of his long working week family life is suffering. It is not easy to juggle career with private life in this profession.

Adrian, Mental Nurse

Adrian trained as a Registered Mental Nurse during which he learned the medical model of mental illness. He administers drugs but is supervised by a senior clinician (usually a Psychiatrist). He gives depot injections to long term mentally ill patients. These are monthly injections into the buttocks or back of the hand. By giving a large dose monthly the patient suffers less needle pain.

Adrian is trained in all aspects of mental illness and carries out therapeutic work in Psychiatric Hospitals and the community. Adrian helps train junior Nurses, a part of his work he enjoys. He is studying for a Degree in Nursing and takes time during the day to study.

*

Adrian's patient Stan has schizophrenia, diagnosed 10 years ago. Stan is able to work full time as medication stabilises his symptoms. Adrian is visiting Stan to administer a depot injection. Adrian sees Stan once a fortnight to support him socially. Some patients will be allotted a Social Worker, Occupational Therapist or Rehabilitation Officer as key worker but as Adrian already sees Stan for depots, the team felt it better to give Stan the reassurance of the same person.

It is Wednesday. Adrian is attending the weekly Team meeting. He has prepared reports on his patients and wants to ask for team advice on two. Anna (Psychologist) wants him to see a new patient, Jessica and asks Adrian to set up a joint appointment. It is common for CMHT members to work together. Adrian has room on his caseload so takes on two clients referred from Primary Care (GP Surgery). He asks Marlene to joint-visit a client who needs social skills training.

Adrian is with his Supervisor this morning in their weekly meeting. He likes to arrange this on the same day as the Team meeting so he can use his case notes for both. His Senior Nurse, Tam, notices Adrian looking stressed. Tam asks Adrian if he can cope with the two new patients he has taken on. Adrian agrees he is taking too much on. The senior works with Adrian to rearrange his diary.

After lunch Adrian calls Mrs Abrahams who has panic attacks. She has recently been bereaved of her teenage daughter and finding it hard to come to terms with her loss. Adrian offers an appointment with CRUSE, a charity specializing in bereavement counselling.

Adrian does not feel well and decides to take the advice of his senior. He cancels a less urgent appointment and goes home. Tomorrow is another day and it is vital for him to retain his mental well being, or he cannot help his patients.

John Jethro, Community Pharmacist

John Jethro is a qualified chemist and prepares some pills himself. He enjoys this part of his work. Most medications are off-the-counter commercial drugs from pharmaceutical companies. John is happiest when customers ask his advice as it makes his work more interesting.

Not many customers realize he is a scientist and probably knows more chemistry than most General Practitioners.

By law he has to be in the shop when medicines are dispensed in case customers ask questions about how medication must be taken:

- with or without food
- number of times a day
- if foodstuffs 'contra-indicate'* with the medicines

   *some foods react with medicines making it ineffective and other foods are dangerous when taken with certain medicines.

9.00am Friday and the shop is about to open. John is late. Sally, one of the assistants, serves a customer with toiletries but the lady wants a specific medication which needs the presence of the Pharmacist. By law, Sally is not allowed to sell this if the Pharmacist is not on the premises. Her customer is annoyed but Sally has to be firm. Luckily, John arrives. The shop is not busy so John retires into the pharmacy to mix tablets. As it is autumn, he decides to buy stocks of influenza and cold preparations as he knows which brands sell well.

After lunch a pharmaceutical representative arrives with samples. Just as the Rep is leaving the telephone rings. The Hospital has a cancer patient who needs a drug and their supplies are exhausted. The Pharmacist they use at another Hospital has been called on an emergency and there is no one else in the locality with a qualification to dispense. John dispenses and hands the package to the motorcycle courier. All drugs have to be accounted for and there is a trace system. John adds the drug to Sally's order. Sally has prepared a list of out of date medicines, which have to be destroyed, and she adds these to the fax she is sending to the suppliers.

6.00 pm and the shop is officially closed. John sees the local drug addicts who have arrived to pick up scrip's (prescriptions). Addicts are prescribed legal chemical substitutes such as methadone which lessen the effects (cramps, hallucinations) when they attempt to give up hard drugs after years of use. Many Pharmacists set aside time outside normal shop hours for this task as they know customers can be upset at the appearance or behaviour of addicts. They need to protect their business interests.

6.30pm and they put on the alarms and lock up. John is looking forward to a lecture he is giving to trainee Pharmacists at the

University. He looks forward to the time that Pharmacists can prescribe and be given public recognition of their chemical training.

Paul Lacey, Psychiatrist

Psychiatrist patients are offered appointments ranging from ½ to one hour, considerably longer than the 10 minutes allotted to GP patients. Diagnosis of mental illness is a longish process and patients have to be allowed time to 'tell their story'.

Paul Lacey deals with what are called forensic cases, which means patients who break the law as a result of behaviours connected with their mental state. He will have on his case list both paedophiles and patients with psychopathic personality disorder. Publicly these people might be reviled, but Paul has to perceive them as patients who need treatment.

*

8.30 am. The list is full and there are appointments in the Psychiatric Hospital as well as community visits to do. First visit is to Gannoway Prison where he is visiting Mackenzie. Mackenzie or Mac is a habitual alcoholic in his 60's who is dying from alcoholic poisoning. Mac has schizophrenia. He stabbed and severely wounded his brother Joe, under a delusion that Joe was an alien. Mac is in prison because there is nowhere else for him to go. The secure hospital 20 miles away has no beds and there are none at the local Psychiatric Hospital.

Paul has a soft spot for Mac who is likeable when his delusions pass. Mac is a good cartoonist and is drawing when Paul enters his cell. The portrait depicts a devil and angel arm-wrestling in grey and blue chalks. Paul persuades Mac to have a depot injection.

Mac likes being in prison because he feels secure and is well fed. He has no home and knows the 'screws' (Prison Officers) well, treating them as family. Mac's family refused to visit after the incident with Joe. Mac does not want to be given parole at his next review as he feels safer in prison. He is likely to commit another offence if released, so he can stay in prison which is his only home.

Next call is the Hospital where Paul is running a seminar. He enjoys doing training. One of his Trainees is convinced a new therapy has cured a long term patient. Paul knows the patient has been having such 'cures' for 20 years but does dampen the trainee's enthusiasm. He suggests his student observes the patient longer. An anxious Mental

Nurse hurries toward him and asks him to see a patient in the next room. The patient is sitting in the room not responding.

Pamela is sitting on the floor, distraught. By gentle questioning Paul ascertains her partner has left, unable to cope with her illness. Now she has financial and housing worries too. Paul offers reassurance and arranges for a Social Worker to call. The Nurse is grateful but embarrassed he had not thought of this solution. Outside the therapy room Paul reassures the Nurse that the obvious is not always apparent, especially when she is worried.

Paul is late for his next appointment, a lady in a manic state. This is a very distressing illness not only for the patient but her family. Marcia is accompanied by her daughter, Ann. During the height of a manic episode Marcia took £8,000 out of her bank account and gave it to a dubious charity. Marcia is extolling the virtues of the charity but her daughter is crying. Ann tells Paul her mother is behind with mortgage payments and likely to lose the family home. This situation is not unusual amongst manic patients as unscrupulous people take advantage. Unfortunately there is no law to prevent this.

Paul is unable to stop Marcia getting deeper into a manic episode. He cannot legally section her, despite the ruinous financial implications, as her actions are not a danger to life. However, he does persuade Marcia to have a Haloperidol injection which will reduce her manic level. After helping Ann get Marcia to bed and asking Adrian to provide social support, Paul leaves. He dislikes patients being cheated, yet knows there is nothing he can do to intervene.

Late afternoon finds him in his office writing case notes and lecture notes. Each week he attends a Journal Club which gives advanced training to Junior Doctors. It is one of the few occasions they can meet with peers during the working day.

On his days off Paul likes to swim and play golf. He finds it hard to fit the work he loves with the responsibilities of a large family (4 children under 9 years). He has to be careful his marriage does not suffer under the strain of the long hours which are a part of his job.

Peter, Psycho Analyst

Analysis is not available on the NHS because of the cost and time involved and patients are usually private. Patients attend from 2 to 4 sessions a week. Each session lasts 45 minutes; this is referred to as the therapeutic hour, as the last 15 minutes is used by the Analyst to write patient notes. Psycho analysts do not write notes in the session as they give full attention to their patient.

Peter has been a Psycho Analyst 10 years. Before starting training, he had to undergo this own training analysis before being accepted as suitable for the training - some 5 more years.

*

Peter takes his dog for a walk every morning to refresh his mind. Peter has three clients today. He is due to see Stella at 9.30am. She sees him twice a week for 45 minutes. Stella has been his patient 3 years and is about to conclude. She referred herself after a very unhappy childhood followed by an unhappy 15 year marriage. During the marriage Stella lost confidence and wanted to work with Peter to find a better future. She wanted to work out why the marriage had failed so if she re-married things would be different.

During these 3 years Peter listened, allowing Stella to work things out for herself. He would occasionally repeat to her what she said to bring her unconscious thinking into her conscious mind, which is how analysis works. Stella told Peter of her dreams during analysis. Through the dreams, which were sometimes violent, they discovered Stella was angry with her deceased father - anger she had been unconsciously directing toward her husband. Peter takes 15 minutes after Stella leaves to write notes.

His next patient is Jester who chose that name, but is a sad man who has schizophrenia. Not many Medics believe schizophrenia can be treated through analysis but analysis was commonly used as a therapy before anti psychotic medication was developed.

Peter is having remarkable success with Jester, who is an intelligent man. Jester's delusions centre on a bizarre circus. Peter had an intuition this circus represented feelings and emotions Jester had been bottling up. After working for months Jester's delusions are reducing and he is beginning to deal with difficulties in real time. As Jester leaves, Peter sees his third client of the day driving up the lane. This is a new patient, Marilyn.

Marilyn is early for her appointment. Peter signals out of the window he has seen her and completes his notes on Jester. Marilyn is a cross at being kept waiting and expresses this by deliberately knocking one of his plants off the stand as she enters, watching for his reaction. He smiles inwardly. Is this how she expresses anger in everyday life? The process of analysis begins.

Peter loves classical music and draws his violin from its case. A little Mozart, perhaps, he muses. He lives a full life. He has learned from experience how important that is.

Anna, Clinical Psychologist

Psychologists treat patients using behavioural or cognitive behavioural therapy. Whilst they train in the medical model (chemical theory of mental illness) they are not medically qualified and do not prescribe.

Anna studied for a Degree in Psychology followed by further training of 3 or 4 years. She became a junior Psychologist and the completed on the job training before being allowed to register as a Clinical Psychologist. Psychologists conduct research and publish clinical papers on the basis of evidence gathered from interaction with patients. They conduct research in the community, for example upon the social effects of mental illness in families.

Anna, like many trainees, had been interested in people from an early age. She had a difficult childhood and an innate curiosity about why people behaved the way they do. It was curiosity which drove her towards psychology. Eventually she came to realize that though psychology held interesting answers it was not a cure for every problem. That aside she enjoyed her time with fellow students and kept in touch with them by attending professional events organized by the British Psychological Society.

*

Jenny (one of Anna's patients) was treated cruelly by her father during childhood and for many years became frightened at work when male bosses criticised her, bursting into tears but becoming embarrassed later. This affected her career. Jenny is making mistakes at work and losing confidence. This is causing unhappiness and triggering depression. Jenny is unaware her childhood experience is connected to her fear of bosses. Anna calls Jenny's behaviour towards men as 'a negative behaviour pattern'. Jenny herself calls it '*the silly way I am*'; though she is aware of what she is doing, she can't stop.

Anna uses cognitive behavioural therapy, a method which helps Jenny understand how her relationship with her father is repeating in her working life. By bringing this behaviour pattern to awareness Jenny can to work towards more productive behaviour.

Anna visits the ward to see long term patients, most of whom have been diagnosed with schizophrenia. There is no cure for this illness but medication controls the delusions and hallucinations. Anna sees her role as improving the life of these patients, helping bring order into their chaotic world. She has devised rehabilitation programmes, carried out by the Occupational Therapist and a Rehabilitation Worker. Simple tasks such as washing, dressing or cooking are difficult for someone with schizophrenia when they are overwhelmed with delusions. A structured day is socially beneficial and reduces anxiety. This is true of many mental illnesses.

After seeing patients and talking to Ward staff about the management of the programmes, Anna returns to her office to write case notes. This is an important part of the work. Notes are required so other professionals can refer to them when Anna is not there.

In the afternoon she goes on a community visit to a patient with severe depressive illness. Sandie should be in hospital, but her husband is adamant he wants her at home. This makes Anna's job difficult, but as the lady has not shown suicidal intent, she agrees. Anna explained why depressive illnesses occur and how they are treated. She has to repeat this information constantly as people under considerable stress cannot take in information.

After 1½ hours, which is a long time in therapeutic terms, Anna drives to her next appointment. She is to train local staff in Behavioural Therapy techniques as their Psychologist is away. Afterwards, she talks to the Team Manager.

She and Social Worker Adrian are visiting a man suspected of sexual abusing his two grandchildren. The man is abusive and aggressive in contrast to his wife, who is weeping. The man admits the abuse but is unable to see he had done anything wrong. '*She asked for it*' he says adamantly; the 'she' in question is 7 years old. Eric calls the police when the man attacks his wife. There is no cure for paedophilia but mental health services have to protect the public. The man will be visited in his police cell by Dr Lacey.

It is the end of the working day. Anna has one more patient, a lady nearly cured of agoraphobia (fear of open spaces). Anna has been working with Patricia for months. It is difficult to imagine what an effort this has been but Patricia shows her delight by giving Anna a present, a paperweight. NHS staff are not allowed to take gifts from patients, but as this is for Anna's desk she accepts.

Alison, Psychotherapist

Alison sees clients for an hour once a week over a longish term of up to a year or longer. Alison helps her client explore their life problems, and help them understand why the same difficulties keep repeating. Alison lets her clients decide on the issue to be talked about in each session. If she feels her client is evading something or dealing with too much at one time, she will bring this to their attention.

Alison was a teacher before deciding in her 40's she needed a change of direction. She went to the library and looked up entry requirements for re-training as a Psychotherapist. Many people decide late in life to train in the therapies and this is looked on favourably, as older therapists bring life experience.

Alison cannot wave a magic wand to make people better. She is a person who has problems in her own life but copes. She likes people enough to devote a career to healing others.

*

Alison is seeing David. David has problems socialising, though he is a highly intelligent man. David finds it difficult to express his feelings when he meets a girl he likes and after a few dates breaks off budding relationships. Then he becomes depressed and angry. This week David tells Alison about a time his favourite pet dog was run over but was unable to cry, although he wanted to.

He and Alison spent the hour talking about other occasions when sad things happened and David was unable to express emotion. Towards the end of the hour David suddenly remembered how as a child he cried when his favourite teddy had been thrown in the rubbish.

For David, the teddy was his only friend but his unsympathetic father had beaten him and told him not to be a baby. Remembering this in the session David began to cry. He cried for ½ hour. Alison asked why he was crying and David said it was the first time he could remember not being punished for crying. They were able to talk about how wrong his father was not to have let David express emotions.

A Psychotherapist sees 4 or 5 patients in a day. This type of work is emotionally demanding.

Marlene, Rehabilitation Worker

Marlene had no formal entry training as in her time Rehabs were chosen for common sense and life experience, receiving on-the-job training. There is now a City & Guilds Certificate in Rehabilitation.

Marlene deals with all kinds of patients, from the 'worried well' to chronically mentally ill patients. She uses judgement to determine what her patients need and how to achieve that end in a friendly, relevant and acceptable way. Marlene must persevere and accept her patient's bad behaviour on occasion.

*

Marlene has a patient called Yvonne with long term depressive illness. Marlene visits Yvonne to take her shopping and has devised a long term programme designed to build Yvonne's confidence. Marlene suspects Yvonne is developing agoraphobia and wants to prevent this. She arranges to visit Yvonne at 11.00am and uses the two hours before this first visit to catch up on housing applications made on behalf of two of Eric's patients. Luckily she has time to visit the Housing Officer and complete the forms.

Today Yvonne is feeling anxious about the untidy state of her home. Marlene helps clear up. This is not her job but it is practical rehabilitation. Her client will benefit from the improved environment. They devise a plan for Yvonne to do small amounts of house tasks every day, including opening post. Depressive illness results in lack of energy and even simple tasks become overwhelming. The plan gives focus to Yvonne's day. Therapists often ask patients to formalize such a plan by signing it, like a contract.

Marlene's second client is Rob, who has been bereaved. Marlene arranges for him to see a Cruse Counsellor who will visit twice a week. Rob cries a good deal and talks in detail about Jen's death. Although Marlene is a trained Counsellor, she cannot deal with Rob herself, as she has recently been bereaved. Mental health workers must be aware of their own mental state and not see patients when they themselves are vulnerable.

Marlene's next visit is to Sal, a teenager who lives in a bedsit two miles from her parents' home. Sal's parents are supportive but Sal is too dependent, visiting them up to three times a day. She wakes them early in the morning by banging on the door. Sal is a pleasant girl whose delusions are fantastical rather than frightening (she sees and hears Angels) but at heart she is lonely and has poor self care.

Today Marlene helps Sal compile a shopping list. An O.T. in training provided a menu which proved too complex for Sal's limited attention span. Marlene and Sal simplified it to foods Sal regularly ate, like readymade pizza and baked beans. Marlene knew Sal would never cook complex meals and would otherwise return to old habits of crisps and chips. This application of practicality versus over expectation demonstrates why life experience is vital in this work.

Marlene's next appointment was Richard, a senior Executive at an Electronic Company. Richard was wary of being referred to a Community Mental Health Team because he thought they only saw 'mad' people. When the G.P. explained he could be visited at home and that this was commonplace, he agreed. Marlene explained to Richard how stress was part of life but that the excessive stress he was experiencing would affect his health, even bringing on palpitations.

By now it was 5.30pm. Marlene wrote up case notes and was about to leave when Esther rang. Esther was a patient with mania. Marlene was fond of Esther - in small doses. Esther frequently rang when she was high and needed someone to talk to. She lived with an aged mother who was deaf. Marlene arranged to see her after the meeting. Esther had not taken her medication so Marlene left a note asking Adrian to check up on her.

Finally, at 6.00pm, Marlene left for the day. Just in time for an evening class in glass making.

Eric, Social Worker

Eric took his Diploma in Social Work several years ago and is now a seasoned member of the team. Many patients on Eric's case book have enduring mental illness (schizophrenia, MDP, OCD). Others are outpatients with short term difficulties. There is still a stigma attached to Social Workers, some folk have an outmoded view that only working people need them, which is not the case.

*

Eric's first appointment is with Susie, who is divorcing and wants social support and help with budgeting. A Court has ordered the sale of the marital home and she has moved with her small daughter into

Council bed and breakfast accommodation, waiting to be offered a flat. Eric is helping her complete Housing Benefit forms.

Susie is distressed at this unfamiliar situation and is worried about the future. Before he leaves, Eric teaches Susie relaxation techniques and leaves a music tape he made for her.

Eric has a couple of free hours so he returns to base. A welcome cup of coffee is followed by a visit to Sam, one of his longer term patients. Eric needs to give Sam a depot injection of drugs which remains in Sam's blood system for a month. They talk about Sam's progress while Eric monitors Sam's mental state. They share news about a joint love of model aeroplanes. Every week after the injection Sam goes to a day centre and Eric waits with Sam until the bus arrives before visiting his next patient, Monica.

Monica is not answering the door. Eric is concerned. He knows she is in, as he saw her walking upstairs as he rang the bell. Eric knows Monica has not been well for some time. She has schizophrenia but has refused depot injections. Eric suspects she has not been taking her medication. Her neighbour recognises Eric. She tells Eric how Monica has been running around her flat late at night, shouting. She is concerned because Monica has become frail and thin.

Eric needs to apply for Sectioning under the Mental Health Act and calls Dr Lacey. He drives to base and gets the necessary papers signed. He returns to the flat with a Police Officer who has a warrant for forced entry. Once the Police Officer has broken in, Eric finds Monica shivering in her bedroom. She has soiled her clothing and the flat is filthy. Eric takes a frightened Monica to Hospital in his car whilst the neighbour arranges to have the flat boarded up. An hour later Monica is in hospital.

Eric is too late for his next appointment and telephones to re-make. His last appointment at 6.30pm is to help Matt complete benefit forms. Eric is thankful this will be straight forward. He and Matt complete the forms and eat a plate of biscuits.

Eric's partner Sally tolerates his erratic working hours, luckily for their marriage.

Jason, Hypno-Psychotherapist

Hypnotherapy and Hypno-psychotherapy are useful for dealing with specific problems of short term duration. Trance states are used by other therapist as an adjunct when relaxation is an issue.

Jason is a former banker who devoted his spare time to Community work. He trained with Cruse (bereavement counselling) and Relate (relationship counselling), doing voluntary work, but soon realised he wanted to build his own private practice. After months considering which course to take, he decided to undertake Hypno-Psychotherapist training, as the School offered weekend training.

Weekend training is common for adults and professionals who are busy during the week. Jason found working and training tiring but knew the future benefits outweighed the not inconsiderable time spent training for his new career. He discovered early on that he was expected to deal with his own life problems first.

*

Nearly 18 months on Jason and has several patients. His supervisor is Mandy whom he visits once a week for around 2 hours, depending on how many clients he is seeing.

First through the door is Andy, who has disabling facial twitches. These are uncommon and distressing. People can be cruel and Andy has been teased about winking not only by children but adults. Jason takes a case history and asks Andy about the twitches (sometimes referred to as *tics*). When Andy tells him about the large number of tics he gets and also the fact he gets angry easily, Jason wonders if Andy does not have simple tic but a form of Tourettes. This needs medical intervention. Andy is naturally upset. He thought a few sessions of hypnosis would be enough. Like many people, he is afraid of Psychiatrists. However Jason persuades him medication might be effective and help with the mood problems. He offers to refer him via a colleague and Andy agrees.

His next client is Daisy who is about to go on holiday but is afraid of flying. She booked the holiday hoping it would give an incentive to overcome her illness and felt guilty because her family longed for a holiday abroad. Jason must work fast as the holiday is three weeks away. After taking a case history he realized the phobia (fear) occurred after a traumatic flight when turbulence caused her flight to crash land on the runway. Unfortunately on her next flight a man had tried to hijack the plane.

Jason spent time reassuring Daisy these coincidental incidents were highly unlikely to reoccur. Jason relaxed Daisy into a hypnotic state (trance or very deep relaxation). First she was to imagine events as they were. Whilst doing this Jason noted her breathing rate rapidly increasing and her fists clenching. In the second trance she had to imagine the same events but with a different outcome, i.e. concentrate on her breathing, rather than events around her. This took Daisy a while but by the end of the hour long session she was feeling better. Jason decided to see her twice more encouraging her to practice. Daisy was able to get on the aeroplane albeit nervously. When there was turbulence she put herself into a trance and coped. Several years later Daisy is still happily boarding planes.

Daisy was able to get on the aeroplane albeit nervously. There was turbulence but she put herself into a trance state and coped. Several years later Daisy is still happily boarding planes with her family. Hypnotherapy and Hypno-psychotherapy are useful for dealing with specific problems of short-term duration. Trance states are also used by other therapists as an adjunct when client relaxation is an issue.

****

Chapter 11
Institutional Care & Support Groups

Content:
1990's Care in the Community
Psychiatric Hospitals
Self Help - Support Groups
Therapeutic Communities

Local newspaper report
'[An] arsonist... who has served 21 years in jail, is on the move today. The man who put him behind bars, Judge... wrote 'In a just Society ... he should not be in prison at all, but in a secure place, where he could be offered and receive treatment.''

1990's Care in the Community
Loneliness. I saw a man from a local Group Home, a house in the community where he had been moved from his long-term home in a now closed Asylum. He was standing on a street corner singing to himself, cradling a pile of incontinence pads held close like a baby in his arms. His face expressed incredible sadness.

Many patients did not want to leave their Asylum homes. Despite the buildings being in bad repair, crumbling and draughty, they had supportive staff and familiar fellow patients. Locals were used to the bizarre behaviours and tolerated it. Although the community was tolerant about patients when they returned to their Asylum at night it was different when the Government decided they must all must live in the community together.

Most patients went to live in communal or group homes, which were houses purchased privately in residential areas. Three or four ex in-patients lived together, compatibility being a matter of luck. The group homes received support visits from mental health workers, one or two a week or more for severely ill patients.

Perhaps not-so-lucky patients were offered bedsits and left to their own devices. There was a spate of petty crime by patients, many of whom had enduring schizophrenia, hoping to be sent to prison in which institution they felt safe. Prisons became congested with seriously mentally ill people.

Care in the Community was based on the premise that the community cares. The reactions of the public ranged from tolerance and indifference to hostility. There was an instance where a so-called sane person threatened to shoot patients about to be housed next door. The authorities bowed to this threat and the patients housed elsewhere.

In an ironic turn around, former Asylums were converted to luxury flats. Where patients lived in wards with peeling-paint and ancient heating systems, the new flats became the luxury dwellings of their former detractors. Many Asylums were pulled down and obliterated from history with not even a street name to acknowledge their passing.

The former asylum St John's Hospital, Stone near Aylesbury, was given listed status but had to be pulled down when thieves stole the roofing lead after security guards were discontinued. The montage shows several views of St Johns. My photographs are available to view in the Buckinghamshire Collection.

Psychiatric Hospitals

The last of the Asylums were decommissioned in favour of smaller Psychiatric Hospitals with out patient departments. With the advance of more effective medication, it was no longer necessary to lock up vast numbers of patients. The Care in the Community Act gave responsibility for day care to Psychiatric Hospitals, leaving a few beds for respite care.

Criminally insane patients were imprisoned in psychiatric prisons such as Broadmoor or the Scottish version, Carstairs. These institutions are run on the lines of therapeutic communities, which are described later. Though there is no effective cure for severe personality disorders, there are effective regimes and treatments which make life more comfortable and humane.

An average 1990's Psychiatric Hospital consisted of several wards for permanent patients, an outpatient clinic for day cases and teaching facilities for junior Psychiatric staff. Rooms were available for therapists (Psychiatrists, Mental Nurses, Psychotherapists and Mental Health Workers) to see out-patients but many patients would be visited at home. There were specialised services such as Art therapy and group therapy.

There was also provision for the so-called 'worried well' (people who did not have active mental illness but were vulnerable due to stress), with training on assertion or stress management, with access to individual appointments with mental health professionals.

Community mental health charities could hire meeting rooms for groups like Alcoholics Anonymous or Cruse and Relate Counsellor training. Many self help groups were run by mental health charities like Mind and Rethink.

Self Help - Support Groups

Many support groups, variable in type and content, were run by a plethora of mental health charities. The fact that patients attend to share experiences does not mean they will like either get on with other folk in the group or find the format agreeable. However, support groups fill a gap between NHS and the private sector. Many patients find them invaluable especially on lonely Bank Holiday weekends.

There are virtual support groups for those with Internet access and computers are provided at main libraries. There are millions of virtual support groups across the world. Americans may be faulted for many things but providing services is not one.

Books and magazines are another form of virtual support. There is nothing like shared human experience to lessen isolation even for those not normally keen on socialising.

Samaritans

Founded in 1953 by Chad Varah, an Anglican vicar who wanted to find a way of alleviating the suffering of the suicidal, this voluntary organisation has branches nation-wide and over 20,000 volunteers. Samaritans went online in 1994 offering confidential email to users in addition to telephone lines. Volunteers from all walks of life undergo a selection process followed by about 30 hours training and six months probation.

Volunteers are selected for life experience and are well supervised. These folk provide free year 24 hour listening to those who are in despair and need an objective listening ear.

Therapeutic Communities

An uncommon form of treatment, Therapeutic Communities comprise therapists and seriously ill mental health patients living together in a special community.

The Community is self-functioning and self-governing and specialises in long-term problems such as addiction, behavioural problems and personality or emotional disorders. Patients are encouraged to take part in the management and hold weekly meetings to talk over difficulties as well as to attend compulsory group therapy sessions.

Each day is highly structured and consists of therapeutic activities interspersed with chores - gardening, cleaning and DIY. Therapies range widely and include some of those not offered mainstream, for example:

- art therapy
- psychodrama
- gardening therapy
- group psychotherapy
- women's and men's groups

There are drawbacks. Therapeutic Communities can be a potential hot pot for exchanging illnesses as well as offering potential growth. However, for those who find it hard to live in a normal community or have been in prison these are undoubtedly the best option, combining understanding, companionship and therapy.

Therapeutic Communities

Patients & therapists live together in a Therapeutic Community. Grendon Undertood for example is a therapeutic community in a prison setting. Relationships are informal and allow patients to learn the skills of community living and social relationships.

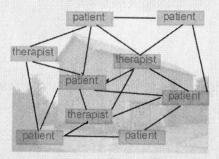

POSITIVE BENEFITS

communal living is natural for the human species
individuals are more self aware in a supportive group
there is more physical and mental security
peer support allows the development of social relationships

NEGATIVE ASPECTS

groups can bully individuals
people develop differently in groups than as individuals
individuals can become institutionalised
        ie unable to live independently outside the group

© author image: an outbuilding at St John's Asylum, Stone

Chapter 12
Case Histories

Content:
Brief Psychotic Disorder - Jane
Depressive Illness - Sally
Eating Disorder - Fiona
Mania - Emma
Obsessive Compulsive Disorder (OCD) - Cynthia
Personality Disorder – Tom
Phobia - Mike
Schizophrenia - Mandy

ALL the following are fictitious people, simplified vignettes which demonstrate classic symptoms of mental illnesses from DSMIV. I have added some complementary remedies for those interested in that area. If you find them realistic perhaps that is a compliment to my creative ability.

In order to make this interesting, try symptom spotting. But, please do not take this exercise seriously - mental illness it is not for lay diagnosis. **If you are worried about symptoms, visit your GP.**

Please also remember, I describe extreme cases in order to highlight symptoms. In real life, no patient has every symptom nor are all the outcomes as portrayed here. There are cases in which treatment is rarely successful or simply not available. It would be dishonest if I did not present this information.

Brief Psychotic Disorder

Brief Psychotic Disorder is the medical term for what is commonly known as *nervous breakdown*. The name describes the condition well; an illness of short duration during which the patient loses touch with reality (psychosis). Psychosis means 'out of touch with reality'. Brief psychosis is of short duration, a fragmenting of the mental processes as a result of overactive chemicals in the brain. This is a temporary and treatable condition, which may never occur again in the patient's life.

111

Psychosis is a feature of many serious mental illnesses such as schizophrenia, but here the delusions are permanent, part of the illness and relieved by constant medication. Sometimes such psychoses come and go, manifesting at times of great anxiety or stress.

What the person sees, hears and feels during a psychosis is real to them but not to those around them. Neither does a psychotic person see a real person but only the object of their delusion. Those who commit murder under delusion are not choosing to kill. It is as if they are in a virtual reality film. Psychotic patients are engrossed in an imaginary world where sensations are heightened. Delusions and hallucinations resemble nightmares such that the sufferer is unable to distinguish night from day and is unable to function normally. Classical art features *day into night* as a theme.

The film *A Beautiful Mind* vividly depicts the delusions of Dr John Nash, diagnosed with schizophrenia whilst he was still at University. Years later, he was awarded a Nobel prize for his economic studies. With the advance of better medication, he was able to live a relatively normal life, continuing his work.

SYMPTOMS:

Physical
- speech unclear
- withdrawal from every day activity
- dishevelled appearance
- agitated

Mental
- delusions –has fixed ideas or beliefs at odds with reality
- hallucinations –sees or hears things that are not there
- inability to concentrate
- extreme fear
- confusion about time orientation ['day into night']

Causes
- major life stress
- following childbirth
- extreme stress states
- after trauma and battle injury
- after bereavement

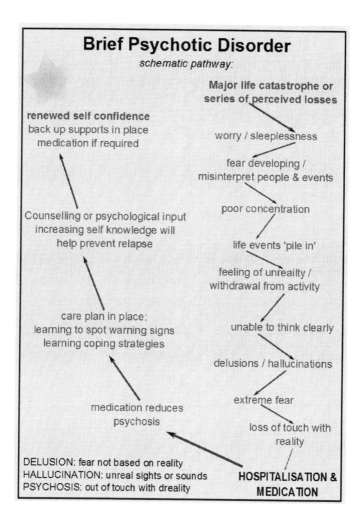

Brief Psychotic Disorder
schematic pathway:

Major life catastrophe or
series of perceived losses

renewed self confidence
back up supports in place
medication if required

worry / sleeplessness

fear developing /
misinterpret people & events

Counselling or psychological input
increasing self knowledge will
help prevent relapse

poor concentration

life events 'pile in'

feeling of unreailty /
withdrawal from activity

care plan in place:
learning to spot warning signs
learning coping strategies

unable to think clearly

delusions / hallucinations

medication reduces
psychosis

extreme fear

loss of touch with
reality

DELUSION: fear not based on reality
HALLUCINATION: unreal sights or sounds
PSYCHOSIS: out of touch with dreality

HOSPITALISATION &
MEDICATION

Attitudes

People are sympathetic to those who develop brief psychotic disorder. They understand it is not the patient's fault. The disorder can be treated with hospitalization and medication. As brief psychosis is common after birth, women tend to talk about it rather than perceive it as something shameful so the perceived stigma is reducing over time.

Cures/ Remedies

- medication to reduce psychotic symptoms
- detainment in Psychiatric Hospital
- supportive counselling

Case History - Jane

'If I had to go through this experience again, I would kill myself. It was like being in hell. I thought 'they' were following me trying to control my mind; everyone appeared to be in the 'plot' even my GP and my husband. I couldn't trust anyone. I went to bed exhausted and woke up sweating and terrified. I was living in a nightmare day and night. If I had not gone to hospital I would never have recovered.'

Jane is 40 and separated after years of marriage. Neither the marriage nor Jane's childhood were happy. She has no family and lives alone. She works full time in a clerical job which she does not particularly enjoy. Jane has few friends. She is not a life and soul of the party type but her friends appreciate her quiet manner and ability to make them feel cared for.

Her friend Joe noticed Jane's answer phone had been left on for two weeks. Although it was customary with Jane not to answer every call such a length of time was unusual. When he called at her flat the curtains were closed and he noticed an upstairs light on, though it was still light. Joe rang Cynthia a mutual friend. Cynthia said Jane had not attended a writing group which was Jane's favourite hobby. Next morning, Joe and Cynthia called Jane's employer who said she had gone in one morning acting strangely and then run off.

Joe and Cynthia called the Police. A warrant was obtained by the police and a Police Officer and Social Worker met Joe and Cynthia at Jane's house. After a delay, Jane answered the door. They were shocked by her appearance. Jane looked terrified, refusing to allow them in.

Cynthia eventually persuaded her to let them pass. The house was in a mess, full of overflowing bin bags, litter and half eaten meals. There was a stench of rotting rubbish. Cynthia tried to hug Jane but she backed off, crouching in her chair, rocking and shouting at someone only she could see. The Social Worker asked Jane a lot of questions. Jane said she had visited her GP and told him a man in the waiting room was listening to everything they said and making notes. Though this was a delusion, it still seemed very real to Jane. The Social Worker took Joe and Cynthia aside and said he would have to detain Jane under the Mental Health Act. Joe asked if he and Cynthia could take her to Hospital. He was aware that, were Jane to be committed (sectioned) she might have difficulties with her employers, who were not sympathetic. The Social Worker agreed. After a couple of hours of coaxing Jane was persuaded to go to Hospital.

Next day when the Psychiatrist arrived, Jane again showed fear. A Mental Nurse gave Jane a tablet which she refused. The Nurse asked Jane why she was not taking the medication and Jane said the Psychiatrist was trying to poison her. Jane's belief was so strong she could not be persuaded otherwise. As Jane become agitated and began thrashing about, a group of Nurses held her down while a sedative was administered.

Cynthia and Joe continued to visit. She was healthier looking, thanks to regular sleep and meals. Jane felt trapped as the doors to her Ward were locked, to prevent very ill patients wandering off. Jane wanted to walk in the Hospital grounds but the Nurses said she was not allowed for her own safety. Days were tedious on the Ward, with little to do. Jane attended some art therapy but was left on her own for most of the day. She could retreat to her room when she wanted and this gave her respite from other ill patients, whose behaviour upset her as she recovered awareness. Released from the stresses of everyday life and work, she slowly began to recover her sanity.

Jane, terrified by her ordeal, found it hard to talk to the Counsellor at first. Cynthia was present at one session, with Jane's permission, and they talked about how she and Joe might support Jane when she was discharged.

Several weeks later, Jane was discharged and offered ongoing counselling at home. She was embarrassed at things she had said and done during her illness, for example, believing the Consultant had been trying to poison her. The Counsellor reassured her that this was a common symptom of psychosis.

A year or so later Jane found a new career more to her liking, with pleasant colleagues and caring employers. She continued her friendships with Joe and Cynthia and eventually was able to talk freely about her ordeal and what she had learned from it. Her symptoms did not return.

*

Depressive Illness

Guilt over the suicide of a relative is extremely common, when in reality there is no blame. Depressive illness is treatable but needs to be dealt with as soon as possible.

Depressive illness is a serious mental disorder, not normal life sadness. Relatives often blame themselves for not spotting signs - but it is hard to detect even for professionals. People with depressive illness are very good at hiding how they feel, to avoid upsetting family and friends. People of all ages and walks of life commit suicide under a delusion their relatives will be better off without them. **Note:** their thinking is pathologically irrational, a symptom of the depression, caused by changes to the brain chemistry. At this stage, it requires hospitalisation and immediate medication.

People worry about what to say and do when a relative is seriously depressed. Telling a depressed person '*pull yourself together*' is as helpful as giving this advice to someone with a broken leg. Psychiatric assessment is the first requirement with continuing human contact and comfort.

*

Depressive illness is common.1 in 4 will be treated for depressive illness at some time during their life. The most unexpected people suffer depressive illness, even 'life and soul of the party' types. Consider the suicide of poor Robin Williams, the American actor, known for his outgoing personality and almost manic cheerfulness. Untreated chronic depressive illness can be lethal, with suicide a strong risk factor.

After Depression

The experience of depression is isolating, frightening & difficult to understand for those who have never suffered in this way. However with insight, suffering leads to new experiences and ideas. Many writers and artists endure mental illness. I wrote this poem whilst recovering from clinical depression triggered by a failed relationship.

Prometheus

Where are the Furies swords that cut so deep?
Where the woman wild with voiceless cries
Denying sleep?
Why does the night hold daggers to my eyes
And rack my heart with pain
Send salty tears run coursing down
In twisting veins.

Why am I denied the calm
When storms subside
Ceasing restless seas of pain.
Oh Lear! Cut out my eyes
And tear my face with Harpy claws.
Let the Eagle rip the liver open wide.
When my body's gone
Will the soul look down
In sorrow and despair.

Alone I walk in darkest silence
Along the highways of the night
And there upon the shore to watch
The crashing waves and restless sea
Scent salty air and hear the curlews cry
And watch the moonbeams dancing light
Reflecting in my eyes.

Depressive illness has more than one cause as described in the symptoms section. It requires psychiatric treatment and medication to rebalance the brain chemicals [serotonin and nor-adrenaline]. This can take a number of months, or years, but relief is usually found within a short time of first taking medication.

The most misunderstood symptom of chronic depressive illness is a suicidal urge. The patient will not be thinking rationally; it is delusional. Suicide notes reveal people saying irrational things like *'you will be better off without me'*. Sadly, some suicidal people take children with them, under the delusion they will be better off 'with God'. All this is highly distressing for those left to deal with the resulting anger, guilt, trauma and shock.

SYMPTOMS

At least 5 of the following must be present almost every day:

Physical
- sleep disturbances (lack or increase of)
- lack of energy
- decrease or increase in physical movements
- changes to weight and appetite (increase or decrease)
- withdrawal from activity and social life

Mental
- persistent low mood (marked irritability in children & teens.)
- tearfulness
- lack of concentration or decisiveness
- lack of pleasure in everyday life and activity
- feelings of guilt or worthlessness
- thoughts or desire of death

Causes:
- changes to brain chemistry
- family history of the illness
- abuse of alcohol or drugs
- loss e.g. bereavement, amputation, job, opportunity, relationship, some precious object
- life events of all kinds

Cures/ Remedies
- medication to supplement brain chemistry

- Electro Convulsive Therapy (ECT)
- Cognitive-Behavioural Therapy (when recovering)
- counselling (when recovering)
- mindfulness or meditation training (when recovering)

Sadness and Depression

The difference between sadness and depression is like the difference between a cold and pneumonia. Depressive illness is an imbalance in brain chemistry which blocks chemicals responsible for well being.

Clinicians use testing systems of which the most well known is the *Beck Depression Inventory* (BDI). This questionnaire has multiple choice answers each with a score. Scores are measured against a scale which indicates severity of illness at the time the form is completed. It only works when the patient is honest answering the questions. Beck's tests the shifting pattern of depression.

People fear being considered weak (particularly males) and try to keep depressive illness hidden, often becoming angry or irritable as a result. Some people believe the illness can spread like a virus but of course it cannot. It is distressing to be around someone who has been depressed a long time but regular contact with friends and family benefits patients, even if they express a desire to be left alone.

Suicidal Urges

Suicidal urges are strong. The patient's inability to do anything about the urge can prevent suicide in the depth of the illness. Suicide more often occurs when recovery begins and patients gain the mental and physical strength to carry out such plans. It is vital that anyone expressing suicidal wishes is taken for assessment. People are not being dramatic, they are expressing a need.

How Long Does Depression Last?

Depression requires support from family and friends as well as medication. After taking anti depressants, there will be some relief within a short period but medication must not be continued. It can take months for brain chemistry to right itself and produce sufficient serotonin. Discontinuing medication too early is likely to result in relapse. There is no set time for recovery which varies from patient to patient. However, it is not instantaneous and may require several weeks for the medication to 'kick in'. Counselling is usually offered at the same time as well as regular monitoring by a Psychiatrist or GP.

Case History – Sally

'It was like being at the bottom of a pit. No ladder was long enough to pull me out. I felt a shadow following me – I called it my Black Shadow. I remember sitting in a chair unable to move but I was still aware of friends visiting and as I began to recover, that comforted me. I could not respond at the time and sometimes I didn't want them there. But all the time I was really saying, for God's sake don't leave me alone. It was the most isolating experience I've experienced. Every day, I had thought how sweet it would be not to wake. Of course, I think differently now.'

Sally reached her 46th birthday. She was unhappy, having suffered periods of depression all through her thirties. These had never been treated, because Sally did not tell anyone how she felt. Once she half-heartedly to a Counsellor but broke off therapy to avoid feeling uncomfortable. Sally was so familiar with her depressed mood that she called it her *Black Shadow*. Giving the illness name as if it were a tangible object is common. Churchill called his depression, his black dog. I called mine, my dark angel.

Sally's mother had a history of depressive illness and died age 46 after an unhappy married life. Her aunt committed suicide. Sally often thought about her mother. She felt her mother's life had been wasted on the wrong man. She was angry with her parents for constantly arguing or not speaking, which spoiled her childhood.

Sally married John, a kind man but who found it difficult to talk. When she was depressed he would anxiously do things for her. He did not understand what was happening to his wife. Over several months Sally became withdrawn. If John tried to talk to her, she snapped or burst into tears. She would sit for long periods doing nothing as the house became dirtier and the washing piled up. Sally no longer had the energy or inclination to make love and rejected John's advances.

John felt rejected. He started an affair. He tried to avoid Sally by going to the pub, sometimes coming home drunk. Her friends could not cope with her suffering. When they visited Sally she sat in her chair not responding. Eventually, they stopped visiting.

Whereas most people would feel alert after a night's sleep, Sally woke feeling heavy and tired. Most of the night she had lain awake thinking repeated thoughts about the worthlessness of her life. In the mornings it took Sally hours to get dressed. Getting out of bed was an effort. She felt more secure, being curled up in bed. Though her bad feelings were still there, it gave sanctuary from what she experienced as a hostile world.

Eventually Sally stopped bothering to get up. Feeling more and more isolated despite the efforts of her partner, Sally decided it would be better to die and started writing a note. Luckily John came in, saw her suicide not and was shocked. He insisted Sally immediately went with him to their GP.

Sally's GP prescribed ante-depressant medication to lift her mood and made an appointment for a Psychiatrist. John was reluctant for his wife to go to a Psychiatric Hospital because he thought only mad people went to there. The G.P. reassured him these places were for anyone with mental health problems. As soon as she was stabilised, and taking regular medication, Sally could be discharged and attend as a day patient.

John asked how long Sally would have to take antidepressants. The G.P. said it might be several months, but he would reduce the dosage as she recovered. Sally would visit a Counsellor to help regain her confidence. The GP wanted John to be involved in Sally's treatment.

Throughout this period, Sally's recovery was erratic. However, she was reassured by staff and regularly tested for mood levels, using the Beck Inventory. At the same time, John found a Counsellor to deal with his own problems. He was given information about relationships and depression and felt less guilty as he realized Sally's depression was not his fault.

As Sally recovered, she and John realized they were no longer in love. Sally wished her mother had divorced, as her feuding parents made the childhood home very unhappy.

Sally started training for a new job as a Nursery Nurse. Sally stayed in the marital home whilst John rented a flat locally. They were able to talk freely for the first time in years.

Sally started to make new friends, although she preferred being at home after her recent traumatic experience. During the next few years Sally did relapse but each time she felt stronger and able to seek help when she needed it. In time the symptoms disappeared.

*

Eating Disorder

Formerly divided into anorexia nervosa and bulimia nervosa, eating disorders are now grouped under a single diagnosis. Anorexic types tend to restrict intake of food whereas bulimics tend to binge then purge (laxatives or vomiting). It is not that such patients do not want to eat; they often crave food and are obsessed by it. The drive to not eat and purge are impossible to control. It is frightening for the patient as well as relatives. The urges stem from the illness, not the patient's rational thinking.

As well as an urge to eat or void, there is a malfunction of self perception. People find it hard to understand how teenagers weighing 6 stones or less think they are fat. It is an illness of perception, called body dysmorphia. Eating disorders affect 1% of the population, usually female but with a growing tendency among teenage boys.

Do you remember being a teenager and thinking you were fat and when you were older re-visiting your photographs and being surprised you were normal size? It's the same mental trick played in the minds of those with eating disorders. Negative perceptions are difficult to shift. Force feeding ensures survival but to cure the illness needs to change the patient's perception so what they see in the mirror reflects reality. It is a very difficult concept to understand, unless you have experienced it.

Eating disordered patients in hospital are cunning about concealing and destroying food even. There comes a stage when their body organs cannot cope with lack of nourishment. A high proportion (25%) of seriously ill eating-disordered patients die from organ failure.

SYMPTOMS

About 2 episodes a week over 3 months of the following:

Physical
- body weight fluctuation
- recurrent vomiting or purging (by patient) or restricting food
- teeth decayed because of stomach acids from vomiting
- menstrual cycles disrupted and may disappear altogether

Mental
- fear of gaining weight (anorexia)
- obsessive about body shape & weight

Theoretical Causes
- history of family problems
- fear of growing up and facing independence
- bullying or teasing at school especially about appearance
- desire to control themselves or their families
- media obsession with body image

Attitudes

Even among medical staff this illness is misunderstood and nurses have historically not been kind. Families are devastated. Imagine seeing your child self-starving but knowing you can do nothing. With new knowledge and psychological methods, the outlook is improving.

Cures/ Remedies
- compulsory hospitalisation with a strict feeding regime
- psychotherapy
- group Therapy
- collaboration between Royal College of Psychiatrists and media to present realistic portraits of human health and beauty

Case history - Fiona

'It seems hard to believe, looking back after 18 months on the ward. I mean, I was literally a walking skeleton. Mum showed me photos they had taken. I weighed 5 stones and all I could see was this out-of-control fat person. Jesus. You know what turned things? It was Janine, my room-mate on the Ward. They said I could say goodbye before the Undertaker came. There was the bed and a rumpled sheet. I thought they'd taken her body but was curious and looked under the sheet. I couldn't stop vomiting. I could see all her bones through her skin. I was terrified. What if I looked like that and didn't know it?'

Fiona walked slowly into the office and smiled wanly. I tried to hide my shock. Just behind the thin skin I could see the outline of her skull, a vague circular blueness, the high points of bone protruding from her thin skin, her teeth mottled. It was at variance with the picture her mother showed me of Fiona at ten; a happy, smiling child.

She noticed my shock and looked puzzled. She was a young woman of twenty six, married, with a kind husband and caring parents. She had a steady job and enjoyed painting and clubbing. She was looking forward to having children and only agreed to see her General Practitioner because her menstrual cycle had stopped.

He took one look, listened to her refusal to go to Hospital, then called a Social Worker. Fiona was sectioned. She was too weak to resist but kept repeating there was nothing wrong, only her periods.

Dr Redding warned me Fiona was low but I've never seen anyone that emaciated still alive. The hardest bit was trying not to stare. I saw her once a week for several months. Fiona hadn't been abused or deprived. She had loving parents, friends, a boyfriend and a good job. She told me these things sitting with her feet curled under her, looking like a waif, often not giving eye contact.

We started to talk about weight. She hadn't minded talking about feelings but the minute I mentioned weight, I noticed her thin hands grip the chair, her tongue darting around her dry lips.

On the Ward, Fiona was weighed every day and when meals arrived one of the Mental Nurses would sit with her, to make sure she did not hide or vomit food. Fiona was cunning like the other eating disordered patients. When the Nurses weren't looking she told me how the plants and toilet cisterns received doses of squashed up food. She even hid food in her slippers, flushing it down the toilet later. Luckily the Nurses were wise to these deadly games.

It was months before I managed to get through. It was after her friend Janine died. Janine was 22 and weighed 4½ stones. Fiona was quiet, subdued. She started saying how sometimes people might see things that weren't right, just, '*sort of narrowing things down a bit*' as she put it. We began to talk more. About magazines and how there were only six Supermodels in the population. We talked about getting older and she said that was scary. We talked on and on, about feelings and this and that. We never talked about Fiona's weight or Fiona's food. We just came to an understanding. One day she blurted out about the rape.

Sadly she split up with her boyfriend. He could not cope with the strain. I discharged her two years later. I remember her waving, walking down the drive to the Hospital, hand in hand with her mother. She was still slight for an adult. She looked elfin-like, with the huge eyes of an African child. But there was a glow about her and a little spring in her step. Of those who entered hospital with her – Jamie, Esther, Sally, June, Marina and Nadine, only Fiona and Marina lived.

*

Mania

Many of our finest creatives (artists, writers, poets) have been diagnosed with mania. Mania is characterised by periods of intensive activity, rapid bursts of energy and irrational thinking. The moods are opposite to those of depressive illness.

The illness can manifest alone or more commonly with depression (bi-polar or MDP). 'High' and 'happy' are not the same thing. There are elements of happiness, extreme happiness even, with in a manic high, but when patient perceives they are going out of control the experience can be frightening. Think of times when you have laughed, loud and long and imagine you need to stop laughing but can't. Your muscles are aching, everyone has had enough but you just can't stop. As a parallel, think of Moira Shearer in the ballet The Red Shoes; the red shoes are haunted and she wants to stop dancing but can't.

Manic people can be fun to be with until the mood swings so high it becomes embarrassing. As with depressive illness, a manic attack cannot be controlled. The brain chemistry is firing at speed and only medication can reduce it. It is only upon recovering that the patient is aware of their destructive behaviour (such as excessive spending or promiscuous activity).

Links to Depression

People who suffer depressive illness are, to a greater or lesser degree, prone to attacks of mania when they come out of low mood. It is almost as if the brain says, that was hellish, so I'm going to make sure it doesn't happen again by becoming excessively happy. But like depression, mania is an illness state, not a choice.

Bi - Polar Illness

This is a common variation, the sufferer going from depressed to manic in varying cycles. The moods swing from one extreme to the other in cycles of varying duration. The swings can be erratic, of long or short duration or with long lengths of time between episodes.

SYMPTOMS
Physical
- increase in energy (psychomotor agitation)
- marked increase in activity levels

- decreased need for sleep

Mental
- patient highly inflated opinion of him/her self (grandiosity)
- very talkative
- lack of concentration
- may indulge in promiscuous activity, or unwise investing

Causes
- imbalance of brain chemistry
- family history of the illness (genetic factors)
- over reaction to recovery from depression
- abuse of alcohol or drugs

Attitudes
Mania is uncommon. People might tolerate what can be perceived as euphoria, unless the behaviour relates to a dangerous situation, e.g. someone trying to jump off a high building in the belief they are invincible or trying setting fire to a building under a delusion.

Radio DJ Kenny Everett was frequently hospitalized for mania, yet was acknowledged as the most creative DJ of his generation.

Kay Redfield Jamison's *Touched With Fire* is an excellent book on the subject of creativity, genius and mania.

Cures/ Remedies
- medications which change the brain chemistry
- psycho analysis - used before the advent of medication
- behavioural therapy

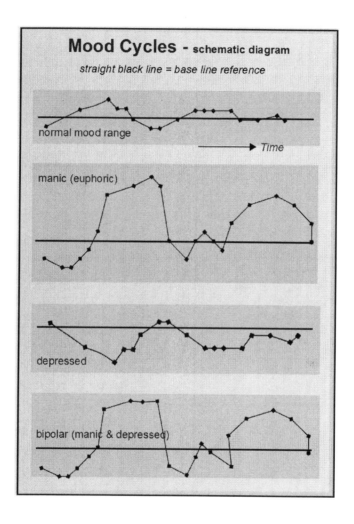

Case History - Emma

'*I've been coming down over the last day or so. I enjoy the mood when it comes on. There's no warning just a buzzy feeling like champagne bubbles in my blood. The world is colourful. Even the grass is brighter and greener. Do you like that, greenier? That's a word I invented when I was high. I feel a tremendous burst of energy and you know I feel I can do anything!*'

'*I went shopping last time*' (she points to her wardrobe, bursting at the seams with colourful clothing). '*Look at that lot! The credit card company was furious. It took months and I'm still paying it off. But wow! I remember how it felt in the shop. Everyone was looking and I was really enjoying myself. God, just like mother!*' She looks uncomfortable and wriggles in her chair.

'*After a few days I get sweaty. I know the mood is overtaking me and I can't control it. My voice gets higher and louder and I grit my teeth but there's nothing I can do. I just jabber on and on and get ideas.*' She looks embarrassed.

'*And I keep picking up men. One night stands. Sometimes more than one at a time. It's great at first then I get uncomfortable. But I start to whoop and shout, and they get scared and leave. I want to sleep but can't and keep pacing the room. I feel used.*' She breaks off into loud sobs. After a minute she brightens and rubs her face.

'*But, well, it's good at the time. The moods are rapid though I get dog-tired. Up then down. Not depressed, you know, but normal mood for me is being down. It's all or nothing. Yes, it's exhausting. I can't stop whatever I'm doing. And the money I've spent! God, I must have wasted thousands on stuff. No wonder shop-keepers love me.*'

'*I call myself Esmerelda when I'm high. Esmerelda* [the gypsy from The Hunchback of Notre Dame by Victor Hugo]. *Do you like it?*' She doesn't wait for an answer but gets excited. *Sanctuary! I imagine myself swinging from the rope into the Cathedral. What fun. The Queen went to the Premier, didn't she? I wanted to meet her. I am sure she would have liked me. I nearly met her at a Garden Party. Gosh, I should have been an actress.*'

She breaks off, fetches a glass of water and a bottle of pills. She opens the bottle and dramatically swallows two.

'*There. I need them but it's hard to remember. It's Lithium. Balances me. Supposed to. Look at that..*' She holds out her hand which is shaking. '*Been like that for years. God, I feel old!*' She looks in the mirror, sighs and plumps down in her chair. Big tears roll down her cheeks.

'*I do feel really, really old. It's like I've lived two lives and not enjoyed either. And I know they make fun of me – think I'm an old drama queen and laugh behind my back. But honestly if they only realized what it is like. I'm scared inside and exhausted*'.

'*I feel like the girl with magic dancing shoes. I can't stop. Oh, sometimes I just wish I was normal, just for a while.*'

She sinks into her chair and I unable to say anything sit and almost feel her exhaustion. I imagine what her relatives are suffering.

*

Obsessive Compulsive Disorder (OCD)
We all check doors are locked before going out but when this gets out of order and becomes obsessive, it becomes a crippling illness. The obsessions [about the thing or idea] lead to a compulsion (ritual or task) to alleviate the obsession. Rituals, like religious rituals, tend to bring comfort and ward off potential disaster. The person is aware of what they are doing but can neither control the action nor explain it.

OCD can be long-standing. Obsessive people are orderly to an excessive degree. It is not common, occurring in only 1.5 to 2% of people in a year. Not much is known about this illness, but it is assumed the causes genetic factors and chemical imbalance. It is difficult to cure although CBT and medication can reduce symptoms.

Obsessions, Compulsions, and Rituals
This unusual disorder has three common elements:
- Obsession – a fixated idea which cannot be stopped
- Compulsion – an uncontrollable urge or belief
- Ritual – rigid procedures in a specific order

Orderliness
People with Obsessive-Compulsive Disorder (OCD) are over organised. They will lay out objects regimentally. It is as if they cannot tolerate disorganisation. The compulsion to make things orderly is not under their control. Neither can they stop before completion of the tasks they set themselves.

SYMPTOMS
Mental – Obsessions
1. persistent ideas – e.g. their house is contaminated
2. Persistent thoughts – burglars are going to raid their home
3. Persistent images – crude sexual imagery

Physical – Compulsions
1. constant hand washing, (sometimes until the skin bleeds)
2. repeated checking and testing of locks and doors
3. constant praying to try to negate guilt feelings

Causes:
- Imbalance in brain chemistry
- Trauma
- Genetic factors

Cures/ Remedies
OCD is treated with medication. There is has no known cure at the present, but symptoms can be controlled with medication and psychological treatment. Patients are given a programme of CBT which reduces exhaustion from doing the ritual. The patient has counselling to help discover the cause of the obsession.

Case History - Cynthia
Walking into Cynthia's home was like walking into a show house. Nothing was out of place, not a speck of dust. She perched on the edge of a rather uncomfortable-looking leather chesterfield wearing a neat navy suit of an old-fashioned kind. Her immaculate hair was lacquered in place, every detail of makeup perfect. Nevertheless as we spoke I noticed her glancing regularly into a large mirror on the opposite wall brushing imaginary stray hairs.

'*I first started,*' she gestured helplessly with her hand, '*this, well, cleaning a year ago. At first I wasn't aware what I was doing. Marjorie, my daily help, kept asking if I wanted to dispense with her services. I asked why. She said there didn't seem need. I told her that the house needed a deep clean and she might have an extra day for the work.*'

Cynthia paused then managed a smile. '*Well, she was honest. After a week, she sat me down and asked me to look. Gradually I took in her meaning. I spent literally all day on my hands and knees rubbing every spot of dirt from the carpet then an hour scrubbing my hands. My hands were raw and the skin between the fingers bleeding.'*

Cynthia sat looking at her hands, then at me. *'It started soon after my husband, Geoff, died. It was a chest infection.'* She paused again and I nodded. She gestured with her hands unable to speak.

'So' I said *'Perhaps you wanted to scrub away memories as if it hadn't happened?'*

'It's m*ore to do with blaming myself, really. As if the cleaning could work magic and bring him back. A sort of ritual.'* She sat thinking.

After a few minutes I interrupted. *'And now?'*

'Now' she said, 'I can't control it. I know what I am doing but I can't help myself.'

At that point a red-faced kindly-looking woman opened the door. Marjorie. I looked at the two women.

'Perhaps Marjorie can be a part of this programme. We will be doing something different to your usual practice Marjorie. It will involve not cleaning and encouraging dirt'.

Marjorie smiled. *'Right ho. Shall we start with tea?'* Cynthia laughed.

*

Personality Disorders

There are many types of personality disorder. The most well-known is psychopathic personality disorder. Murders committed by psychopathic serial killers make highly saleable news. However, there are other types of personality disorder which are amenable to therapy, although there is no cure.

Like any other mental disorder, not everyone presents for treatment, unless a criminal act brings someone to the attention of the authorities. Many pathological people live isolated lives in the community – though, of course, not every isolated person is pathological.

There are potentially negative personality traits in everyone (cruelty, greed, goading, anger), but most people develop morals or conscience to prevent these traits getting out of hand. However, patients with severe forms of personality disorder, such as psychopathic personality disorder, do not have the capacity for conscience. Hard to understand, because even professionals do not know where 'conscience' is sited within the brain. However difficult it is to perceive, psychopaths do not have the <u>capacity</u> to understand what they are doing is wrong.

This is not only a genetic condition but driven by upbringing. Recent evidence seems to point this way. A family history of cruelty or abuse is one pointer. These patients have anti-social behaviour patterns ingrained in their genes. From among this group of patients come the wife or husband murderers and batterers; unable to control impulses. The dreadful acts they commit leave little public sympathy. For Psychopaths, their fate is lifetime incarceration in prisons for the criminally insane – Broadmoor or Carstairs. Yet, they are people too, very ill people whom society has abandoned with little hope of 'cure'.

Where do they go? What do they do for a living? For those on the very edge, the dirtiest jobs, the most dangerous, ones where human contact is not a daily feature and they can hide away.

Others who are less ill might have difficulty holding down a job and suffer enormous anxiety. I do not wish to be downbeat, having heard positive things from a relative of a patient, but they can be difficult as neighbours and frustrating for professionals.

SYMPTOMS
These disorders are divided into types each with a characteristic.
- individual behaves in a markedly different way to others
- experiences problems over a wide range of behaviours
- the condition is long standing

Physical
No marked physical symptoms

Types
- anti social – shuns people and society
- avoidant - inhibited
- borderline – impulsive; difficulties in forming relationships
- dependent – submissive and clinging
- narcissistic – self obsessed
- paranoid - distrustful
- psychopathic – highly destructive; unaware of their illness
- schizoid – withdrawing and detached

Causes:
- Genetic factors
- Dysfunctional home life from early age

Cures/ Remedies
- no cure
- training in impulse control / social skills in therapeutic communities
- medication can control some symptoms
- hospitalisation
- Electro Convulsive therapy
- psychotherapy
- cognitive-behavioural therapy

Case History – Tom

'Never been married, me. Been on me tod since I were a lad. If you'd told me I would be alone at 50 in a place like this– grim ain't it? I'd have topped myself. Thought about it, often.'

He drags deep on his roll up and blows smoke at a ceiling cracked and yellow with ooze. An iron bedstead covered in grubby bedding sags in a corner. A utility wardrobe and dressing table with cracked mirror and two wooden chairs, the ones we are sitting on, are the only other furniture.

'I don't really know why you're here. Yea, it's alright, as long as you don't stop too long. Can't stand company. I expect they told you that.' He drags and coughs. *'What was it like? Working? Ah. Couldn't settle. One job after another– stores, janitor, on the track, van deliveries, day labourer. Used to clear the suicides off rail tracks for extra in one job. Don't bother me. But there's always some cocky bastard or lout gets to me in the end and we fight. I dunno'.* He seems puzzled, rubs his chin and stares at the floor.

'Wanted to stay on the railways. I hate changing jobs. I'm getting on a bit now. Week here, month there, whole year once. Always in the end there's one. I deck 'em or run at 'em. Get me cards. Always the same. Parents? Pop was ex army – Corporal. Corporal Punishment I called him.' We share the grim joke. He laughs then coughs.

'Believer in the strap he was. [vernacular}.. he was. Friends? Na. No one was allowed. Mother? Timid bitch. Mousey. Didn't think much of her. Love?' He laughs bitterly. For a second I think he is going to cry but he controls it, spits and drags on the wet end of his roll-up.

'He used to land her one regular. Stop him? What for? That's what a wife's about, ain't it? When I was older I landed her one meself.'

'As a kid? Never one for games, never joined in. Wanted to– but, it's hard, you know. I used to watch how the others did it – sort of sidling up then getting in the game. You know what kids are. Cruel little bastards. They'd run off if I got up to bash 'em.'

He laughs harshly. *'I was known for bashing, hitting out hard. Proud? I'll say– it was the only thing I had, me fists. Dad would have been proud.'* He shows a tinge of regret. *'Well, he died see? He never knew. You going? Well, come again mebbe - if I'm in.'* He coughs as follows me to the door.

As I walk down the drive I see him watching from the other side of the grubby net curtains. I know he will never admit it, but he dreads the years ahead. He knows something is wrong but doesn't know what to do about it. No one ever taught him. He is too proud to ask. I know he won't let me in regularly. He'll always find some excuse. Occasionally he might, when his loneliness gets unbearable. He might jump in front of a train, as he says he will. He believes he has no one to turn to – that's how he sees it.

*

Phobia
Phobias are excessive fears about objects, things or situations. They are fears or anxieties about anything – going out, an animal, blood and needles, flying. They prevent the sufferer living a normal life. This condition is fairly common, occurring among about 10 – 11% of the population. Phobias start out specific i.e. fear of a single item, then fear of other things which resemble that item, then to encompass a range of similar things.

SYMPTOMS
Physical
- No physical symptoms

Mental
- excessive or unreasonable fear of object, thing, or place
- avoidance of situation where they would have to face fear

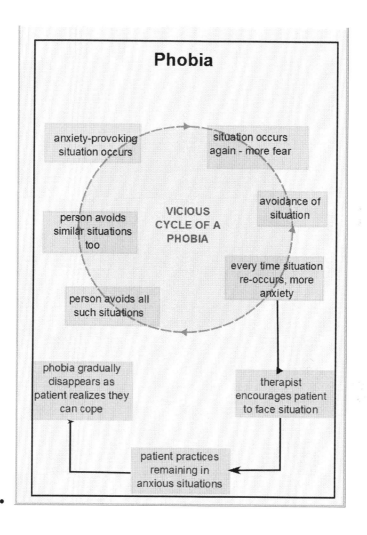

Phobia

VICIOUS CYCLE OF A PHOBIA

anxiety-provoking situation occurs

situation occurs again - more fear

avoidance of situation

person avoids similar situations too

every time situation re-occurs, more anxiety

person avoids all such situations

therapist encourages patient to face situation

phobia gradually disappears as patient realizes they can cope

patient practices remaining in anxious situations

daily living is affected to a marked degree
- the fear is of long standing

Common Phobias
- Agora – fear of open spaces
- Arachna – fear of spiders
- Blood/infection – fear of being contaminated
- Claustro – fear of being in a confined space
- Obsessional Compulsive Disorder
- Post traumatic Stress Disorder (PTSD) –after major accident
- Situational – fear of a situation e.g. flying, spiders, blood
- Social – fear of social situations

Causes
- excessive reaction to negative incidents connected with phobia
- worsening of an existing fear – e.g. fear of spiders
- reaction to loss – e.g. leading to excessive fear of dying
- reaction to incident which occurred in distant past

Cures/ Remedies
- behavioural therapy
- psychotherapy
- cognitive-behavioural therapy

Phobias are treated using behaviour therapy or systematic de-sensitivisation. The therapist encourages the patient to face the situation they are avoiding, but in a controlled way over several weeks or months. One of the talking therapies might be useful, to discover the root or source of the phobia.

Case history - Mike
'I'm sorry I couldn't answer the door. It's getting worse in the last few weeks. Then, I could have got to the garden gate without faintness coming on. How long? I've been confined in the house for 8 months. I last went out with Mary [his deceased wife] for the sales.'

Mike is neatly dressed, his house is bright and clean. He has moved his bed into the lounge and is living in one room.

'It's odd. If you'd told me a year ago I would be afraid to walk outside my own front door I would never have believed it. Neither

would Mary.' He pauses, remembering. *'It began after Mary's funeral. I got out of the car and looked at the trees – started to feel faint. The trees seemed to come in on me. I put it down to sadness. It went off alright. Plenty of our friends turned up. After, we walked to the cars and I felt very dizzy. I was glad to get inside.'*

'After that, it was a succession of things. At first, it was just going to town. It's three miles and I usually drove us. We would have a bite in a café halfway - so I did the same – on my own. The dizziness came back and a bit of anxiety. The first time I rushed back to the car then drove home and it was ok. A few times after that, I had to leave the Supermarket. I was at the check-out when I just had to leave. I can't tell you why, it was a sort of panic.'

'After that it got worse gradually. I had to shop locally. At least I could leave without anyone noticing. And me a man! I was so embarrassed. I always thought this was a woman's thing.'

'Well, eventually I could only get to the gate before this wave of anxiety came. I had to turn back. I'd tell myself it was ridiculous but it made no difference. Every time I panicked, that made it worse next time. I thought if I stayed in the house it would wear off. So I found a home help to do my shopping. I moved everything in this room so I could avoid going out. Sort of nest, really.'

He looks embarrassed and says, with a voice tinged with anxiety, *'Is there any hope I'll get over this? I couldn't bear being confined like for the rest of my life. It's almost as if I'm in a coffin like Mary.'* He bursts into tears.

We persisted for several weeks starting with him walking halfway up his drive. I walked behind him until he was able to get in his car. Eventually, he could do the journey alone, while I waited in the house.

After that he agreed to go for bereavement counselling and things improved from there.

*

Schizophrenia

Schizophrenia is a misunderstood even among medical people, who argue about its disparate symptoms. It is nothing to do with split personality, as is commonly believed. Hallucinations and voices do not always manifest as destructive or evil. They can take the form of religious images, cartoon characters or even banal voices. The unexpected nature of the disturbances, the fact they cannot be controlled, and that they seem to happen outside the mind, renders confusion or even terror in the patient. Artists with schizophrenia are highly creative. Many people live (relatively) normal lives, providing they take regular medication for symptoms. There is as yet no cure.

Schizophrenia is marked by perceptual disturbances, delusions and hallucinations which appear real to the patient but cannot be seen by anyone else. In this way, it can be frightening for both patient and observers. Visual and aural (hearing) disturbances interfere with how the patient perceives the everyday world. The symptoms are disparate and do not manifest at the same time or in the same way. Patients can either display no emotion or excessive emotion.

The film *A Beautiful Mind* depicts the moving story of American mathematician and economics expert Dr John Nash, who developed schizophrenia in his teens. This was before the invention of drugs which control the symptoms. Dr Nash was treated with ECT. Although he never recovered fully, nevertheless he married, had a son and was continued working at mathematical problems, eventually winning a Nobel Prize. The film cleverly demonstrates the delusions and hallucinations that are a hallmark of the illness and I particularly recommend it to new professionals, relatives and carers.

Pre-medication, chronically ill patients were confined in Asylums under constant observation. Now most patients live in the community. Patients with schizophrenia need to continuously take antipsychotic medication, which reduces the delusions and hallucinations.

Schizophrenia in the Headlines
There are a tiny number of people with schizophrenia who fail to take medication and slip through the net of continuous monitoring. Murderous acts are committed by such persons when there are slip ups in legal systems put in place to protect the public. Although such crimes are heinous, it is important to remember these are very ill patients (forensic patients) under the influence of powerful delusions; they are not inherently evil. **More crimes are committed by sane people than by mental patients with schizophrenia or psychopathic personality disorder**.

About 1% of the population is affected by schizophrenia, which first manifests during adolescence, occasionally in middle age.

Diagnosis and Cultural Factors

This illness needs careful diagnosis. Disturbances of vision and hearing can be drug induced. Some cultures are tolerant of factors which in Western culture would lead to a diagnosis of hallucinations and delusions:

- religious ecstasies; seeing spiritual images or 'speaking in tongues'
- ancestors appear to the living to advise them – certain native cultures
- spiritualists claim to communicate with the dead – for them, visual and verbal spirit manifestations are normal

Stigma

Schizophrenia carries huge stigma, the result of sensationalist press I mentioned above. The social effects of schizophrenia are devastating. Patients unable to hold down a job or access social support, are likely drift down the social scale.

In the 1990's, many ex-Asylum schizophrenia patients were imprisoned after committing petty crimes, as a result of being unable to cope with community life. On parole, many committed another offence to be 'put back inside'. Prison life provided the stability and regimentation they required to reduce stress. This tendency was not discovered until prisons became overcrowded with ex-mental patients.

SYMPTOMS

Symptoms must be of at least 6 months duration.

Physical

Patients may show signs of a lack of personal self care

Mental

- delusions – persistent irrational thoughts
- hallucinations – seeing or hearing things that are not there
- speech can be meaningless (word salad)
- no feelings are apparent
- behaviour disorganised or non-existent (catatonic)

Types

- Catatonic– rigid, repeated actions, no stimulation [rare]
- Paranoid – one or more powerful delusions of extreme fear

Catatonia

Now relatively rare, catatonia stupefies the individual in a permanent comatose state. I remember a lady in a Scottish Asylum who sat in the same chair for years, taking meals on her chair and never speaking or moving. A student nurse made considerable efforts to talk to her and the woman responded, only to sink back when this nurse left.

Paranoid

A type of schizophrenia where delusions (false beliefs) are paranoid, a kind of extreme fear. This form can be dangerous if voices suggest the patient commits murder and the patient is not taking medication and being constantly monitored.

Confusion with Psychopathic Personality Disorder

Paranoid schizophrenia can be confused with Psychopathic Personality Disorder. A Psychopath is born without conscience and is unable to distinguish morally. Someone with schizophrenia is able to make such distinctions but acts under delusions which mask reality.

Causes

- generally attributed to one or more of the following:
- family history of the illness
- traumatic childhood/ family events

Treatment

- medications which change brain chemistry
- behavioural therapy, in conjunction with medication
- living in a Therapeutic Community

Schizophrenia is incurable at present but can be controlled with medication. Medication alleviates the psychotic symptoms. However, under the influence of delusions, patients may believe that their medication is poison and refuse to take it or refuse treatment. It is these patients who become psychotic without careful monitoring who might become a public danger – very few in number.

Case History - Mandy

Mandy is an intelligent girl of 26, diagnosed with schizophrenia age fifteen. She lives alone in a small flat and receives irregular visits from her parents and a once a week visit from a Rehabilitation Therapist. After her breakdown she had to leave her Business Studies course, because she was unable to cope with the study. Her boyfriend left her when she was diagnosed and since then she has had no relationships.

'Of course I feel sad about not being able to work, only in a sheltered scheme. The images are intrusive and sometimes the voices are so loud I can't concentrate. I know I will never do the thing I set out to do, Business Management and that makes me sad. I want to be ordinary but I know there is no cure. It took years to accept that.'

'How did I know something was wrong? I didn't; my parents did. I started shutting myself off, I don't know why, except it was difficult to concentrate and I had fuzziness in my head as if there was cotton-wool in my brain. One day I was on a boat on the Thames looking over at the buildings on the other side. A sort of gash appeared in the sky as if it was a painting and someone had ripped a piece of it out, and there were bizarre figures in the rip. I couldn't make it out. I turned to tell my friend and when I told her I saw this horrible shock on her face. She couldn't see it, only me. That really scared me.'

'Then things got worse. I started hearing voices. I couldn't see their bodies but they were very real. No one else could hear them. I assumed they could at first, like the picture thing, but couldn't bear the reactions when I told people, so I kept it to myself. I was just so lonely. My College work suffered. I had been working hard for the exams – too hard. It was impossible to concentrate with these weird things. I was getting mad but trying to make out I was OK.'

'One day I heard a voice saying the boy next to me was going to kill me. I turned to look at him. I could see his face changing. His face started to melt. Apparently, I grabbed an art knife and tried to stab him. That's when they called someone and I was taken to hospital.'

'It was a relief to talk about the visions and the voices. The Doctor seemed to understand, as if it were an everyday thing. I suppose it was to him. Anyway, it made me feel better. Less scared.'

'I asked him if I was mad and he said that madness was a term ignorant people used to describe something they couldn't understand and were frightened of. He said I had schizophrenia and that it could be controlled with medication.'

'I told him I was really scared, that I didn't mean to harm that boy and I didn't want to be locked up. I asked him if I would be put away and he said that as long as I took the medication things would be fine. He said someone from the Community Mental Health Team would visit me regularly and make sure everything was OK.'

'I sort of got very lonely, especially as my parents rarely visited. I know they were upset but I think they were frightened too. I suppose it's easier for them not to come. They couldn't cope with me at home, sitting and talking to voices. I think mum's sister had this too, so I suppose it brings it back to them.'

'Tom, the boy I tried to stab, visits. I felt really guilty but he knows I didn't mean to hurt him. And the voices haven't come back since I started taking the pills. He doesn't mind the flat being messy. I can't get it together to clean often as I get confused. I kind of hope he visits more often. We like to do art together. Maybe we can get together an exhibition. That would be really cool.'

*

Chapter 13
Social & Complementary Approaches

Content:
Social Interpretation
Community Care in Primitive Cultures
The Balanced Personality
Stages of Life
Complementary Practitioners
Aromatherapy/Massage
Reflexology
Art Therapies
Reichian Therapy
Chiropractic/Osteopathy
Crystal Therapy
Spiritual Pursuits
Yoga

The following **do not refer to psychotic symptoms** or any severe symptoms of mental illness, which should be treated with medication and/or hospitalisation. Complementary medicines are mostly un-researched but there is anecdotal evidence some are effective in reducing stress levels. Episodes of mental illness can become more frequent or worsen with high stress levels, and stress reduction is useful for carers and family as well as patients.

There are many charlatans in medicine and the complementaries, so be cautious, especially if you are distressed or desperate for a 'cure'.

*

This brief outline describes alternative ways of viewing and treating illness across different cultures, including so-called 'social constructs' of R D Laing.

If I asked you to describe different ways of getting into a locked house, you might come up many alternatives; use a key, break a window, take the putty out of a window, climb a fence, shin up a drainpipe. Some might be effective, others destructive or dangerous.

How you eventually to get in would depend upon circumstances. For instance, if there was a fire and there were children at the windows. Likewise, there are many ways of alleviating mental illness.

Research proves there are effective treatments other than medicine for relieving the stress, which is a feature of living with mental illness. I will describe stress in more detail in the chapter following.

There is anecdotal, as well as research evidence, showing some complementary treatments reduce stress, induce relaxation and reduce fear. For those with mild to moderate depression, anxiety and other trauma, holistic theories can work well.

*

Social Interpretation

The social theory of mental illness holds there is no such thing as mental illness but only problems of relationships between people living in communities.

Given love, support and understanding the theory goes, people thrive and are tolerated no matter what behaviours they display. Under these circumstances there will supposedly be little anti social behaviour (so goes this theory). Read the writing of Psychiatrist R D Laing who wrote extensively on what he called 'the myth of mental illness.'

Largely disregarded today, Laing is nonetheless educative reading for the serious student of mental illness. There are some parallels with therapeutic communities (described in another chapter) but such communities treat, rather than deny, the symptoms of mental illness. These communities house those with more serious mental health conditions, such as personality disorders.

*

Community Care in Primitive Cultures

In so-called primitive cultures where ancestors are revered, what we term psychotic symptoms are perceived as manifestations of kind, ancestral spirits, who have come back from the afterlife to help the community solve problems. Those who show signs of seeing visions or hearing voices are not hospitalised, but looked after and revered within the Community.

*

Harmony of Mind, Body, and Spirit

Holistic therapists teach that mental, physical and spiritual health (mind, body and spirit) are interdependent. Treatment of one has a beneficial effect upon the other. This balancing of mind/body/spirit results in health and harmony and stable communities (see diagrams)

Imagine you have a cold; does it affect how you feel and think? However, if you are well and the sun is shining does that affect your mental state? It is possible to be physically well and mentally unstable, disabled yet cheerful, physically sound but sour. In holistic therapy, this is perceived as an imbalance in one of the three systems.

Yogis have proven that mind and spirit can transcend physical circumstances, if regular spiritual practice is combined with physical exercise.

*

The Balanced Personality

Refer to the diagrams. Mind, body and spirit each contain different aspects of human existence:

- Mind – relating, suitable occupation, identity, ability to relax
- Body – physical health and appearance
- Spirit - ability to perceive beauty, art, spiritual experience

A balanced person functions harmoniously, operates effectively in their community and copes better with traumas.

*

Stages of Life

There are rites of passage in all primitive cultures. At certain critical times, certain rituals stages have to be successfully completed, before the seeker can successfully move to the next stage. In Western culture, we would perceive stages of life something like this -

- birth
- age 5 – going to school
- age 13 – puberty
- aged 18 – entering adulthood
- age 40's – mid life
- age 80's – old age
- ++ - advanced old age

We all recognise *puer eternis* or eternal youth, the man who never grows up, or the spiteful gossip who lives to a lonely old age.

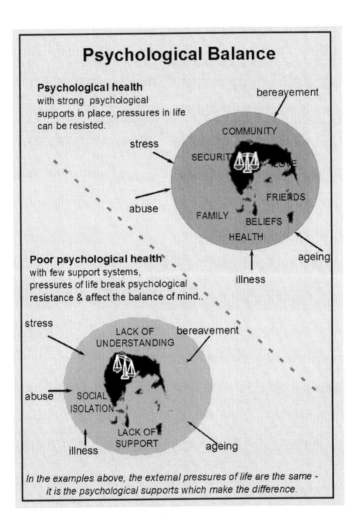

Psychological Balance

Psychological health
with strong psychological
supports in place, pressures in life
can be resisted.

bereavement

stress

COMMUNITY

SECURIT   LOVE

FRIENDS

abuse

FAMILY   BELIEFS

HEALTH

ageing

Poor psychological health
with few support systems,
pressures of life break psychological
resistance & affect the balance of mind..

illness

stress

LACK OF
UNDERSTANDING   bereavement

abuse   SOCIAL
ISOLATION

LACK OF
SUPPORT   ageing

illness

*In the examples above, the external pressures of life are the same -
it is the psychological supports which make the difference.*

In primitive cultures, these difficulties would be perceived as a failure to pass the ritual tests of the previous stage. In some cultures youths of a certain age spend months in the wilderness living off their own resources. At the end of the allotted period, if they successfully complete the rituals, they are allowed to re-join the tribe. They will be welcomed with feasting and ceremonies.

In Western culture rituals are less likely to be physical challenges as dressing up, consuming food and alcohol and receiving congratulatory cards and gifts. Those who do not 'pass' still receive gifts (unlike the unfortunates of the tribes..) but might be quietly taken to a therapist.

A Therapist's task in 'stage of life' therapies, such as Jungian Analysis or Freudian Psycho-Analysis, is to help the client out of the stuck stage. Jungians (followers of Carl Jung) specialize in the important passage through the middle years towards maturity (individuation).

*

Complementary Practitioners

There are more complementary therapies than I have room for in this brief chapter, including the interesting Humour Therapy Clinic set up in the USA by Dr Patch Adams, whose appeal for staff received huge response from Doctors in the US. The movie, Patch Adams, explores Patch's story.

From creative writing and art therapies through Eastern philosophy (Chinese medicine, reflexology) to what has is now mainstream (acupuncture, herbalists, aromatherapy, chiropractic) there is a therapy to suit every philosophy.

In the East there is a saying, when the pupil is ready a suitable teacher emerges. One of life's curiosities is, how often this happens.

*

Aromatherapy/Massage

Aromatherapy is a body massage. The Therapist uses scented natural plant and oils to treat specific problem areas. Plants are the forerunners of 25% of medications we use today. Those synthesised in laboratories assure parity (quality) and considerable research has gone into testing for specific symptoms. In the West we discovered this recently. The

Chinese have known it for thousands of years. Aromatherapy is very relaxing. Once the body is relaxed, the appropriate oils seep deeply into the body and the mind begins to drift. This is good therapy for those who do not like talking about problems.

Aromatherapy provides caring, physical contact without the stress of being psychologically naked. For the shy, masseurs (male) and masseuse (female) are good with strategically placing towels so clients do not feel embarrassed.

*

Reflexology

A similar therapy, for those who do not find physical contact easy, is Reflexology. This therapy is a dry massage using talcum powder on the feet or the hands.

Reflexology works on the principal that the body has meridian lines running through it in vertical lines, each line connecting areas of energy. Pain occurs when there is a blockage along one of the lines which correspond to the body organs the line runs through. The Reflexologist's job is to find areas of blockage and release them through massage, thus restoring harmony.

Reflexology has been used in China and Egypt for thousands of years. A famous tomb of a physician has a painting depicting a scene of reflexology. The patient says '*do not hurt me*' and the practitioner replies '*I shall act so that you will praise me*'. The practitioner is depicted working on his patient's toes.

The theory of meridian lines and balance underlies much of the Chinese medicine system, which works on harmony or Tao of body and mind.

*

Art Therapies

Originally considered fringe, art therapies are now offered on the NHS. In art painting therapy, the patient is given media (crayon, paint, chalk) with which to draw. The idea is not be to create a technical masterpiece but to express emotions. When the piece is finished, the Therapist discusses its meaning with the patient.

There are many art therapies; poetry, reading, psychodrama. Patients in psychiatric hospitals are encouraged to take part in art therapy. Psychodrama involves the client or patient acting out incidents from

148

their past, as if in a play. Interpretations and alternative endings are explored in intense but enlightening sessions.

The only difference between art and art conducted as therapy is that the latter involves interpretation. Certainly writing, drawing, and reading are excellent ways of de-stressing, whether or not they are formal therapy.

*

Reichian Therapy

Reichian therapy is less commonly practiced than it used to be. Wilhelm Reich proposed that during times of mental torment the body locks, preventing the patient moving properly. If the body is unlocked, through Reichian massage, the body returns to harmony and is released from mental tension.

*

Chiropractic/Osteopathy

Chiropractic restores health through manipulating the spine. The aim is to re-align joints which become misplaced through bad posture and freeing nerves which are trapped. It is a similar theoretical stance to Reichian Therapy.

Often when someone is stressed or in crisis, they hold themselves in; hunch, cringe, curl. Now that a large proportion of the population work with computers, posture easily becomes bad through poor siting of equipment. Driving can also seriously misalign the body particularly the neck and spine.

Less gentle, but none the less as effective, is osteopathy. An osteopath makes sharper physical adjustments which can be disconcerting to the beginner.

As well as physical muscular release, these therapies are beneficial in reducing stress and general tension.

*

Crystal Therapy

Natural minerals are beautiful to look at but this therapy proposes that crystals emit vibrations which can be used to heal various aspects of illness. Each type of crystal supposedly works on a specific wave length and heals a different problem.

Not a therapy I recommend from personal use but there is an aesthetic pleasure looking at and handling these minerals. Do not spend large amounts on crystals at healing conventions; you can purchase them more cheaply online.

*

Spiritual Pursuits

Books on Taoism or Buddhism are not the dry tomes you might expect and contain enlightening information. Sufi tales make very interesting reading. These are a kind of allegory. Taoists are renowned for their peaceful demeanour and sense of humour.

The Miracle of Mindfulness by Thich Nhat Hanh (pronounced Tich Nat Han) describes the simple daily practice of mindfulness or full awareness. This practice makes the most mundane tasks enjoyable. I can personally recommend this. Mindfulness is now popular among NHS practitioners.

Any genuine religious practice brings spiritual relief, but needs to be practiced sincerely. Each sect has their own prayers, bible or meditation methods and some use song, but all are uplifting, when experienced in groups of like minded people. The value is in sharing experiences. Beyond words and touch, spiritual practice is good for anyone with mental turmoil, particularly those who find physical or social contact difficult.

*

Yoga

For those who prefer something physical there is Yoga, a watered down Western version of the incredible exercises practiced by Yogis (spiritual teachers) in India.

Yoga is exercise and meditation in one and promotes physical and mental health whilst also promoting suppleness of body. One 91 year old friend of mine (now sadly deceased) remained supple, thanks to taking up yoga at the ripe age of sixty four.

There are many schools of yoga, some very physical and consisting of complex postures, others less so. A form called hatha is gentle and teaches breathing techniques.

*

Carers and the family of mental patients are often neglected, though they have stressful lives. Spiritual practices and complementary therapies should not be underestimated for their positive effects in the relief of stress, but also for social connections.

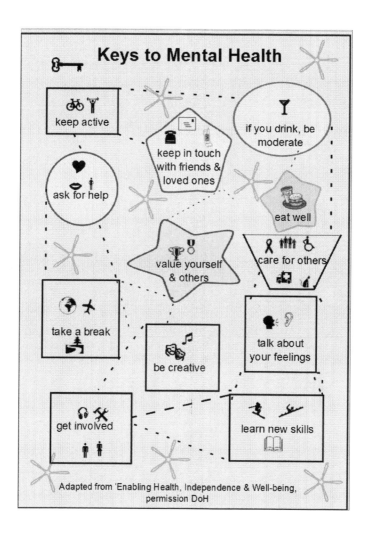

Chapter 14
Stress

Content:
The Meaning of Stress
Physiological Reactions
Stress in Everyday Life
Coping Strategies - brief overview

Stress is a necessary part of life, but excessive stress results in unpleasant symptoms. The chemical causing these symptoms is called Adrenalin. Many people who attend A&E Departments with suspected heart attacks are often suffering adrenalin palpitations. But anyone worried about symptoms is recommended to seek medical advice in the first instance.

*

Patients with enduring mental illness, as well as carers and family, develop high levels of stress. It is not easy living with mental illness, let alone coping with stigmas. People can be intentionally or unintentionally cruel or say irrational things. Coping with these factors will undoubtedly raise stress levels. Understanding stress is therefore a vital part of mental health education. Yet, it is an often neglected area.

The Meaning of Stress
Stress is present in all vertebrate animals. Stress is a state of readiness for action, which allows animals to react to their environment and survive. Without stress, they (and we) would die. To understand what stress is, we need to go back in time to the first men in the Stone Age.

Fight and flight
These people were hunter-gatherers, living on wild fruits and animals. They lived in caves, places also inhabited by lions, bears and other fierce creatures. Everyone, animal and human, was bent upon survival. Survival was, and is, the strongest instinct in all animals.

Now, these Stone Age cavemen were confronted every day with a single purpose; kill, eat and survive. Unfortunately, the animals they relied on for food had the same purpose. And that is where the symptoms of what we call 'stress' come in.

Man, confronted with beast, had two choices; run or fight. If others were hunting with him, the animal was smaller or he had a throwing weapon, he would fight. If the animal were large, he was alone or injured, he would run. Nature gave him a wonderful way of 'knowing' the best choice; we call this instinct. Instinct developed over millions of years as those who adapted successfully survived and those who did not, died out.

Stress

As well as instinct, there had to be a system allowing muscles to react instantaneously to a command; 'run' or 'flee'. This system developed over millions of years, as the fastest and fittest hunters survived and the others, unfortunately, died out. More stress was good!

Let us turn to the word 'stress' and how this fits in with our Stone Age hunters. If you look at the original meaning of 'stress', it gives a clue. My 'Shorter Oxford Dictionary on Historic Principles' (impressive, eh?) describes the original meaning of stress as:

'*[subjecting] a person to force or compulsion*'.

This does not mean attack, but a mechanical force which enables us to move. It is easy to demonstrate. Sit in a hard chair then try to get up, without tensing your muscles. It's impossible. Stress is the tension, or propulsive force, which enables the body to move from one place to another. Simple as that.

But modern useage has imbued the word stress with different meaning. My Chambers Concise Dictionary describes stress as:

'*physical or mental overexertion*'.

So what is a normal reaction has been tagged with pathological meaning. That is why people think of stress as a bad thing, rather than normal reaction to situations (think Stone Age hunters). Before describing the difference between normal stress and 'pathological' or modern over-stress, let's look at the body's physiological responses – what stress was designed for.

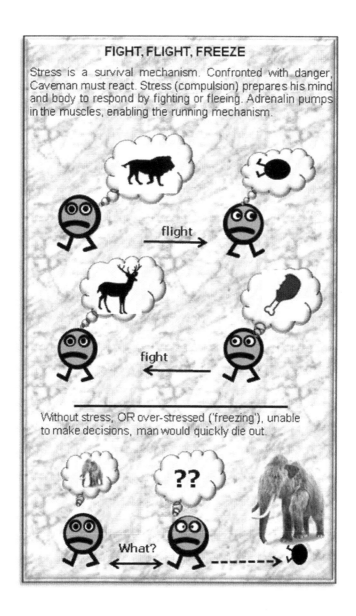

Physiological Reactions

Refer to the diagram on the next page. As well as our hunter, let's imagine an Olympic runner at the start of a race.

When the runner moves from a standing start, a hormone called adrenalin pumps into the muscles when the 'run' signal is sent from brain to muscles. The eyes widen, allowing the runner to focus on the finish line. The breath quickens and deepens. Over time (as the race continues) the breath regulates, adapting to the individual and allowing maximum oxygen to enter the lungs.

If the runner has not done a sensible thing and used a lavatory before the race, faecal matter and urine evacuate, allowing the body to lighten for maximum power. Again, this is normal adrenaline reaction.

There are many other normal reactions to Adrenalin, and I have listed some of them on the following diagram. Think back to a time you were 'stressed out' (colloquial). Compare your physical reactions then to those listed in the diagram. There are many books on the subject which give a more comprehensive list, but you will find the reactions are almost identical. In other words, Adrenalin is the causal factor in both cases; 'normal' stress and modern pathological stress.

The first lesson is, that what is happening is quite normal, even though it may appear alarming to those not in the know.

Freezing

Occasionally, we might go into freeze or 'rabbit in the headlights'. There are few studies on this phenomenon, though it has been recognised as a normal, if rare, reaction to stressor stimuli.

It is thought this freeze instinct stems from the animal behaviour of 'playing dead', an alternative safety mechanism. Some insects do not fly off but imitate their surroundings by way of camouflage.

Though it seems counter-intuitive, these methods seem to work in nature. If you think about it, people who stand up to a bully i.e. neither run nor fight, often induce him/her to give up.

Modern Human Stress

Modern man has no longer a need to fight animals, nor to freeze and stare them in the face. Our food comes from supermarkets and our life spent in offices or factories, not jungles or forests or caves filled with the cries of strange beasts. But, we have not evolved to the stage where Adrenalin is no use.

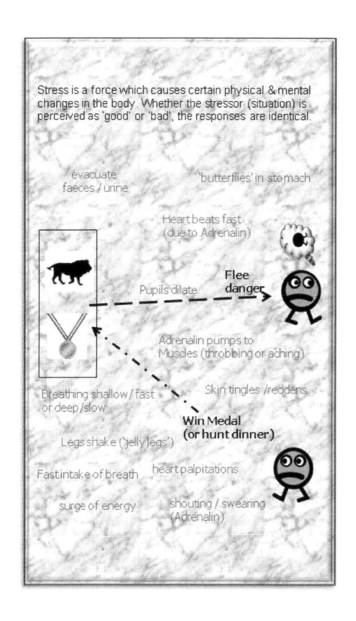

Stress is a force which causes certain physical & mental changes in the body. Whether the stressor (situation) is perceived as 'good' or 'bad', the responses are identical.

evacuate faeces / urine

'butterflies' in stomach

Heart beats fast (due to Adrenalin)

Pupils dilate

Flee danger

Adrenalin pumps to Muscles (throbbing or aching)

Breathing shallow / fast or deep / slow

Skin tingles / reddens

Win Medal (or hunt dinner)

Legs shake ('jelly legs')

Fast intake of breath

heart palpitations

surge of energy

shouting / swearing (Adrenalin)

What if you were about to cross the road and a car came rushing round the corner. What if you turned round, to be confronted by the school bully or a particularly nasty Manager? Offices and factories and living in communities are just as difficult to live in, in their way, and there are times we still need to run, or fight, or freeze..

Stress in Everyday Life

But in everyday life, what happens when Adrenalin floods the system? What happens when we can't run, but must sit at a desk in an office and act as if things are 'normal'? That is when Adrenalin is a nuisance. We need to appear calm and collected, yet our physical reactions show the world we are not. We get headaches, strange cramps or aches, our heart feels as if it is bursting. We might think we are going to have a heart attack or some dreadful illness or disease has come upon us.

Untreated, excess stress reactions can lead to illness. Panic attacks are the result of excess hormones flooding the system. Left untreated, excess stress CAN lead to heart attack, migraine, blood pressure – as well as leading to maladaptive behaviours, like over eating, excessive drinking or drug taking. Though the stress has not CAUSED these illnesses, our reactions to stress, untreated, might LEAD to such illnesses.

So, although stress is a part of daily life, excess stress reactions, left untreated, can lead to illnesses and mental ill health. When stress is reduced, the body chemistry will return to normal – guaranteed.

Coping Strategies – brief overview

This book is a neither a diagnostic manual nor intended for self help but I will list a few coping strategies used to treat mild to moderate stress conditions. Re-visit the section on complementary medicines. Many holistic therapies can be used to reduce excessive stress, but are not generally available on the NHS. They are mostly unregulated and can be expensive.

When evening class season begins, get a list of Local Authority courses, which are cheaper than one-to-one sessions or personal therapy. Many useful techniques can be self-taught from books or tapes. Stress reduction classes are widely available through GP surgeries, by referral. There are plenty of self help websites too. I have listed some resources in the Further Reading at the end of this book.

Apart from the usual relaxations of exercise, walking, passive exercise (TV, movies, games), reading, there are many techniques taken from Eastern practice which have been proven, either by research or anecdotally, to be beneficial in reducing excessive stress.

Creative Visualisation

This method is easily self taught and a kind of self-meditation, based on Eastern techniques. The book 'Creative Meditation' by Shakti Gawain is easy to follow. Creative visualisation involves sitting in a quiet, comfortable place, imagining a beautiful scene. It could be somewhere imaginary, somewhere you have been on holiday or business, or an image you enjoyed from a photograph, book or website. Background music helps, but music needs to be relaxing and repetitive. There is plenty of such music online and some garden centres stock relaxation CD's.

Meditation

Many Buddhist centres offer courses of meditation training, either for a donation or at nominal charge. Meditation is a very old method of relaxation and has many forms, but the method involves sitting or standing quietly, focusing on one aspect, perhaps the breath or an idea or image. The meditation master or leader helps students keep focus, which is the most difficult part of all meditation techniques. There is also a type called walking meditation; unlike normal country walking, the meditator focuses on a single object.

For those used to rushing about or frenetic exercise, meditation can be difficult at first and requires a lot of regular practice. But time and energy devoted to this practice leads to harmony, a calmer life and an increased sense of well being with greater energy.

Mindfulness

Mindfulness is an ancient Buddhist technique, now commonly used in the NHS for stress relief. It is proven effective. The book by Thitch Nath Han is the definitive work and should be available online.

Mindfulness is performing everyday tasks, even mundane ones, with concentrated awareness. Even washing dishes becomes an act of meditation when carried out in this way. A mindfulness student concentrates on every action, focusing on small detail, for example, saying to them self, or out loud, 'As I wash this dish, the water feels silky and warm against my skin.' The student learns to marvel at each fresh sensation, allowing the mind to explore the focus as long as possible, before moving to the next; perhaps 'now I notice the whiteness and translucence of this plate.'

Mindfulness focuses on the inner world, allowing everyday life and concerns to melt into the background. It teaches a sense of wonder and wellbeing, and an appreciation of the detail which frequently eludes us in modern life. During mindfulness, time seems to pass slowly and time awareness improves.

The practice of Mindfulness, like any exercise, is difficult at first but pays dividends for those who pursue its teachings.

Tai Chi

Tai Chi is a soft martial art practiced widely in China but now popular in many countries. Masters of Tai Chi were fighting experts and overthrow opponents by turning their opponent's energy against them. The movements are thought to strengthen and balance inner organs, working along similar principles to the hard martial arts, such as Judo or Karate.

Tai Chi is particularly popular among older people. You do not need to be physically fit to practice Tai Chi, and it improves physical and mental health, breathing, balance and co-ordination.

Tai Chi resembles a slow dance, viewed from the outside. It can be practiced individually or in groups. Tai Chi is a series of movements, which flow one to the other in a harmonious ballet-like motion. The movements each have a meaning and are easily learned.

Affirmations

An affirmation is a short, to-the-point verbal saying or quotation, which can be read quietly or spoken aloud by the practitioner, when they are alone. Affirmations are widely used by complementary practitioners to improve patients' confidence or sense of wellbeing.

Verbal affirmations are shorter and can be adapted from quotations or written specially for the occasion. They can be written in fancy manuscript on cards and pinned to a wall or mirror where they will be viewed daily – not publicly but by the user. Affirmations can also be written on small cards to carried in a handbag or pocket, then taken out in a quiet place to be read (not aloud!) for emergency use.

Examples

Look at the quotations in the following chapter. I will give a couple of examples of how a quotation can be adapted into an affirmation and then one specially written affirmation.

1. For someone always seeking approval:
'The worm that destroys you is the temptation to agree with your critics, to get their approval'
'Hannibal' Thomas Harris
AFFIRMATION: 'I do not need approval. I trust myself at all times.'

2. For someone who doubts they can do something:
'Words do not just reflect reality, they create reality.'
'The Silva Mind Technique' José Silva
AFFIRMATION: 'I will do (xx) despite feeling anxious.'

3. AFFIRMATON: 'I will write a book, starting right now.'

Useful Affirmations

Here are a few I have collected over the years and some of my own.

Community and Responsibility

'Where one member suffers, all the members suffer with it'
St Paul

'Our smallest actions may affect profoundly the whole lives of people who have nothing to do with us.'
Somerset Maughan

'The worm that destroys you is the temptation to agree with your critics to get their approval.'
'Hannibal' Thomas Harris

'I am a part of all that I have met,
Yet all experience is an arch wherethro gleams
The untravelled world whose margin fades forever
When I move.'
'Ulysses' Alfred Lord Tennyson

*

163

Death and Survival

'Things are both more trivial and more important than they ever were... the nowness of everything is absolutely wondrous.'
Dennis Potter – shortly before his death from cancer

'Whoso can look on death, will start at no shadow.'
Greek saying

'When you hear that the individual with the warmest heart and deepest piety ...ended in a gas chamber, then you either go and hang yourself immediately or you have resources within yourself that survive such a moment.'
Viktor Frankl

'If you have built castles in the air--- put the foundations under them.'
Thoreau

'Words do not just reflect reality, they create reality.'
'The Silva Mind Technique' José Silva

'The war broke out... the world of nature was unaffected.. flowers still bloomed, even butterflies still continued their migrations.'
'Sweet Thames Run Softy' Robert Gibbings

'Think work and act; don't sit here and brood amongst insoluble enigmas.'
Henrik Ibsen

'Without work all life goes rotten; but when work is soulless, life stifles and dies.'
Albert Camus

'Cheshire puss, would you tell me which way I ought to go from here?'
'That depends a good deal on where you want to get to'
'Alice in Wonderland' Lewis Carroll

'It's not wise to make life into hell by anticipating things that may never happen, nor, for that matter, by anticipating those that most surely will happen.'
Robert Falcon Scott

'The great human law—that merit is in the long run, recognised and rewarded.'
'Up from Slavery' Booker T Washington

Happiness
'It is activity which renders man happy.'
Goethe

'She was considering in her own mind, whether the pleasure of making a daisy chain would be worth the trouble of getting up and picking the daisies.'
'Alice in Wonderland' Lewis Carroll

'Life is a chain made up of many diverse links. Sorrow is one golden link between submission to the present and the promised hope of the future.'
'The Prophet' Khalil Gibran

'I would not have missed this time of poverty. One learns to value simple things.'
'Memories Dreams and Reflections' Carl G Jung

*

Hope
'Where there is much light, there is a darker shadow.'
Goethe

'Bear and endure; this sorrow will one day prove to be for good.'
Ovid

'There are certain times in our lives when we find ourselves in circumstances that...seem to weigh us down. They give us not only opportunity but impose the duty of elevating ourselves.'
Goethe

'Above the cloud with its shadow is the star with its light.'
Victor Hugo

'The sun is always shining above the clouds.'
Marianne

'He said not 'thou shalt not be tempested' but 'thou shalt not be overcome'.
Julian of Norwich

*

Maturity

'To be magnanimous, mighty of heart, is to be great in life; to become this increasingly is to advance in life.'
Ruskin

'If you wish a wise answer, you must put a rational question.'
Goethe

'We may measure our road to wisdom by the sorrows we have undergone.'
Bulwer Lytton

'If you do not err, you do not gain understanding.'
Goethe

'He who does not see the angels and devils in the beauty and malice of life will be far removed from knowledge, and his spirit will be empty of affection.'
Khalil Gibran

'Everything can be taken from a man but one thing: to choose one's own way.'
Victor Frankl

'So many out of the way things had happened recently, that Alice began to think that few things indeed were impossible.'
Lewis Carroll's Alice

'To underestimate oneself is as much a departure from truth as to exaggerate one's powers.'
'Sherlock Holmes' by A C Doyle

'A man may conquer a thousand warriors, but the greatest of all is he who conquers himself.'
Chinese saying

*

Mental Health

'The mind is ever genius in making its own distress.'
Oliver Goldsmith

'The mind is its own place, and in itself, can make a heaven of hell, a hell of heaven.'
John Milton

'The world considers eccentricity in great things (to be) genius; in small things (to be) folly.'
Bulwer Lytton

'A mind that is free sees that dependency on (anyone) breeds fear.'
Krishnamurti

'Who am I then? Tell me that first, and then, if I like being that person I'll come up; if not, I'll stay down here till I'm somebody else.'
Lewis Carroll's 'Alice'

*

Relationships

'Where people are tied for life, 'tis their mutual interest not to grow weary of one another.'
Lady Montagu (1930's)

'If you would care to dislike a man, try to get nearer his heart.'
J M Barrie

'He who terrifies others, is himself in continual fear.'
Ovid

'I could give you a basket of roses, but they would only fall; I give you the flower of friendship, the most lasting gift of all.'
Marianne

'A man, sir, should keep his friendships in constant repair'
Dr Johnson

'But if the while I think on thee dear friend, all losses are restored and sorrows end.'
Shakespeare

'I am a part of all that I have met. And a part of me belongs to all I meet.'
Tennyson

'If there's a secret to being loved, it lies in not having to be loved.'
M Drury

*

Strength and Tenacity
'The glory is not in never falling, but in rising every time you fall.'
Bovee

'Believe that each new day that shines on you is your last'
Horace

'Where difficulties are overcome, they become blessings'
Traditional Saying

*

Anticipating Success
'The seeds of today are the flowers of tomorrow.'
Unknown

'Success is to be measured, not so much by the position that one has reached in life, as by the obstacles which he has overcome while trying to succeed.'
'Up From Slavery' by Booker T Washington

'Realize, don't theorize.'
Paul, former patient of Marianne

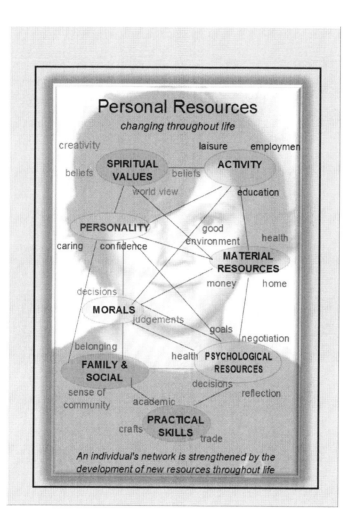

Personal Resources

changing throughout life

An individual's network is strengthened by the development of new resources throughout life

Further Information

Freud, along with many others, believed books give a unique insight into the working of the mind. There are few academic books which portray the human mind in torment and bliss, but a rich seam is to be found in poetry, fiction and film. It's no use recommending books I haven't read so forgive me if I miss any gems – and tell me!

There are many support groups but publishing national help-line numbers creates a frustrating trail to local groups, the details of which are always available in libraries. I hope the following prove enjoyable reading to whet your appetite for further study.

*

ART WITH MEANING
Psalms from the Bible
Pure poetic expression of the joys and sorrows of living.

Selected Poetry of Kathleen Raine
A fine metaphysical poet – I love her work.

Any paintings by William Blake
An artist who successfully portrays madness, suffering and the human spirit.

The Plains of Heaven by John Martin
One of his religious themed paintings; sit by it and enjoy the depth of experience it expresses.

Beyond Bedlam Published by Anvil Press
Very moving poetry by patients of Bethlem Hospital.

*

BOOKS ABOUT LIFE
The Road Less Travelled by Scott Peck
Self improvement, by a giving, generous man.

The Prophet - Khalil Gibran
A beautifully written prose poem about the meaning of life.

The Tao of Pooh by Benjamin Hoff
An allegory about life, based on the children's characters.

Jonathan Livingston Seagull by Richard Bach
An allegory about daring to express individuality.

The House at Pooh Corner by A A Milne
A children's book with many lessons about friendship and acceptance.

Tono Bungay by H G Wells
A life enhancing book with an allegory of how greed, success and failure finally bring peace to a man's life.

The Door in the Wall by H G Wells
A short story about belief and perceptions.

Be Still and Know - The Miracle of Mindfulness by Thich Nhat Hanh
A Taoist monk gives some very practical tips of how to enhance mundane experiences.

*

BIOGRAPHIES/DIARIES
Anne Frank – the Diary by Anne Frank
The moving and often amusing experiences of tragic Anne Frank, written shortly before she died in a concentration camp.

*

MENTAL ILLNESS
Dibs, in Search of Self by Virginia Axline
How a lost child was brought back to the world by a Psychotherapist.

Touched with Fire by Dr Kay Redfield Jamison
Manic depressive illness – and creativity. A gem.

Hallucinations by Oliver Sachs [RIP]
A fascinating book about unusual hallucinations and delusions by the Psychiatrist and master story teller.

DSM IV* Diagnostic & Statistical Manual of Mental Disorders
THE psychiatric diagnostic manual as used by the Medical Profession.

172

Final Exit by Dr Derek Humphry
The controversial suicide manual written by a Doctor who helped his terminally wife end her life.

The Man Who Thought His Wife Was a Hat by Dr Oliver Sachs
Psychiatrist Sachs portrayals aphasia, an illness which prevents patients translating what they see.

The History of Bethlem by J Andrews, J Briggs et al
A primer for those interested in historical treatments.

*

FILM
Shine
The true story of garrulous pianist David Helfgott, who overcomes nervous breakdown to marry and play concerts in public.

Patch Adams
A doctor dons a clown outfit and proves that laughter is as powerful a cure as any medicine.

Awakenings – based on the book by Dr Oliver Sachs
The intensively moving portrayal of a Psychiatrist who successfully woke patients who had lain comatose for years after suffering encephalitis during the Influenza pandemic after the First World War.

*

WEBSITES
The following are the links to the key facts pages for a range of mental illnesses.

Anxiety and phobia
http://www.rcpsych.ac.uk/mentalhealthinfo/problems/anxietyphobias/anxiety,panic,phobias.aspx

Bipolar disorder [formerly manic depressive psychosis]
http://www.rcpsych.ac.uk/mentalhealthinfo/problems/bipolardisorder/keyfactsbipolardisorder.aspx

Community Mental Health Teams

http://www.rcpsych.ac.uk/mentalhealthinfo/treatments/communityteams/keyfactscmhts.aspx

Depression
http://www.rcpsych.ac.uk/mentalhealthinfoforall/problems/depression/depressionkeyfacts.aspx

Eating Disorders
http://www.rcpsych.ac.uk/mentalhealthinfo/problems/eatingdisorders/eatingdisorderskeyfacts.aspx

electro convulsive therapy [ECT]
http://www.rcpsych.ac.uk/mentalhealthinfoforall/treatments/ect.aspx

Obsessive Compulsive Disorder [OCD]
http://www.rcpsych.ac.uk/mentalhealthinfo/problems/obsessivecompulsivedisorder/ocdkeyfacts.aspx

Personality Disorders
http://www.rcpsych.ac.uk/mentalhealthinfo/problems/personalitydisorders/personalitydisordersfacts.aspx

Schizophrenia
http://www.rcpsych.ac.uk/mentalhealthinfoforall/problems/schizophrenia/schizophreniakeyfacts.aspx

Psychotherapies
http://www.rcpsych.ac.uk/mentalhealthinfo/treatments/psychotherapies.aspx

Spirituality
http://www.rcpsych.ac.uk/mentalhealthinfo/treatments/spirituality.aspx

MENTAL HEALTH CHARITIES
American Internet Mental health
http://www.mentalhealth.com/

Bipolar UK [formerly Manic Depressive Alliance]
http://www.mdf.org.uk/

Depression Alliance
http://www.depressionalliance.org/

MIND mental health charity
http://www.mind.org.uk/

Rethink [formerly the National Schizophrenia Fellowship]
http://www.rethink.org/

Anxiety UK [includes info on OCD]
http://www.anxietyuk.org.uk/about-anxiety/anxiety-disorders/obsessive-compulsive-disorder-ocd/?gclid=CM6EyrbvwK0CFUVTfAod_06DAw

OTHER

School of Pharmacy web site
http://www.rgu.ac.uk/subj/pharMacy/pharMacy.htm

The story of Phineas Gage
http://www.guardian.co.uk/science/blog/2010/nov/05/phineas-gage-head-personality   and http://brightbytes.com/phineasgage/

*

GLOSSARY

A

acupuncture	Chinese treatment, for re-balancing energy
agoraphobia	fear of open spaces
anaesthetic	drugs rendering patient impervious to pain
analgesic	pain killing drug
ancestor worship	culture of venerating dead relatives
anorexia	eating disorder, restricts food intake
anti psychotic	drug reduces symptoms of psychosis
anti social	difficulties in socialising
arachnaphobia	fear of spiders
archetype	character in personality (Jungian theory)
aromatherapy	body massage with aromatic oils
asylum [Asylum]	place of refuge. Institution for insane
autonomous	automatic systems e.g. breathing, heart
avoidant	characterised by 'avoiding' situations

B

beck	rating for depressive illness
behaviour therapy	therapy aimed at modifying behaviour
Bethlem Asylum	2nd oldest Hospital in UK; former Asylum
bi-polar	mental illness; depression & mania
blood phobia	fear of blood or needle infection
borderline	mild personality disorder
brain chemistry	chemicals of brain
brief psychosis	short episode of hallucinations, delusions

BPS	British Psychological Society
Broadmoor	Psychiatric Hospital for criminally insane
bulimia nervosa	eating disorder of purging and vomiting

C

Carl Jung	founder of Analytical Psychology
Carstairs	Scottish equivalent of Broadmoor
case history	patient's psychological and physical state
catatonia	mental state characterised by total inertia
catharsis	'purging'; 'letting go' of negative trait
CDPOM	drug dispensed on handwritten prescription
checking & testing	part of compulsive disorder 'checking'
chemical transmitter	way brain chemicals are distributed to cells
Chiropractic	manipulation; re-aligns skeletal system
Cinderella	Archetypal innocence rewarded
claustrophobia	fear of confined spaces
cognitive-behavioural	changing behaviour patterns
compulsion	urge to carry out a certain act or ritual
contra indicative	reacts badly with chemicals (drugs)
counselling	one of the talking cures
crimes of passion	crime committed during intense emotion
Cruse	charity providing bereavement counselling

D

delusion	ideas perceived as real but are imagined
dependent	personality disorder - clinging to another
depressive	mental illness - hopelessness and sadness
DSM	Manual for diagnosing mental illness

E

ECT	Therapy for chronic depression
EEG	electro-encephalograph of brain activity
empathy	understanding of personal situation
episode	period of mental illness
extraordinary	[perceptions] - taken as signs of madness
extrovert	outgoing, confident personality

F

False memory	unreal, imagined events
Forensic	criminal mental illness e.g. PPD

fragmenting of mind - psychosis

G

genetic	cause attributed to inherited genes
grandiose	delusional belief
group [therapy]	treating several patients in group setting
GSL	general sale list; drugs at a Pharmacy

H

Herbalist	therapist prescribes herbs
histrionic	disorder of exaggerated emotions
holistic	therapy including mind, body, spirit

I

imbalance	lack or excess of chemicals in synapses
insight	ability to understand psychological situation
integrative	from more than one school of thought

interpret	help patient gain insight
introvert	inward looking personality

J

Jungian	Analyst of the Jungian tradition.

L

leucotomy	psychosurgery, cutting frontal lobe of brain
lobotomy	see 'leucotomy'
Chancellor	Senior Judge in English Law

M

mania	intense moods/ frantic behaviour
MAOI's	monoamine oxidase; antidepressant
medication	drugs to alleviate symptoms of illness
MIMS	manual of drugs, used by GPs
molecule	smallest particle of a particular chemical
muscle	drug to relax muscles before surgery
mutagenicity	ability of a drug to affect organs

N

narcissistic	personality disorder of extreme self interest

O

obsessional	illness of obsessions and compulsions
old lag	one who commits crime to stay in prison
Osteopathy	therapy involving manipulation of spine

P

panic attack	sudden fear without warning
paranoia	extreme fear
paranoid	form of schizophrenia
Patch Adams	American Psychiatrist; uses humour therapy
persistent	unwanted ideas which will not go away
phobia	extreme fear
placebo	inert medication, part of drug trial tests
POM	prescription-only drugs
pow-wow	palaver; tribal meeting, to resolve problems
Primary Care	GP Surgery / practitioners who work there
psyche	of the mind. After Greek Goddess Psyche
Psychiatrist	Doctor qualified in Psychiatric Medicine
psychodrama	therapy 'acting out' scenes from patient's life
psychology	science of the study of human behaviour
psychomotor	state of frantic activity as in manic episodes
psychopathic	personality disorder absence of 'conscience'
psychosis	intense fear; mind unable to function
Psychotherapy	talking cure; patient develops 'insights'
PTSD	stress disorder after trauma, accident
put away(verb)	Victorian euphemism - lock in an Asylum

R

rhetorical	questions asked to trigger a debate
ritual	ceremony to mark life changes e.g. middle age
Royal College [of Psychiatrists]	UK body of Psychiatrists

S

Samaritans	organisation to help suicidal people
scapegoat	animal /person sacrificed to expiate sin
schizoid	personality disorder; detached
schizophrenia	fragmentation of personality
School	method of training - 'school of thought'
screws	[slang] Prison Warders
sectioned	[slang] detained under Mental Health Act
serotonin	chemical transmitters in the brain
social misfit	Victorian term; social nuisance
social phobia	fear of social situations
split	two personalities in one person

T

talking cure	talking to effect a cure
tic	involuntary muscle movement, Tourettes
toxicity	level of toxin or poison
trepanning	cutting piece from skull; primitive surgery
tricyclic	antidepressant; structure 3 ('tri') rings
trip	[slang] hallucination induced by drugs

V

voodoo	witchcraft of a cult in Haiti

W

witch mark	C16th; area of no feeling
word salad	babbling as in some forms of schizophrenia

INDEX

Analgesic, 82
Anti Psychiatric Movement, 33, 45
Anti Psychotic, 82
Antidepressants, 82
Behaviourists, 33, 40
Bethlem Asylum, 23, 31
Blind' Or 'Placebo' Tests, 76
Brain Chemistry Imbalance, 69
Brief Psychotic Disorder, 111
Care In The Community, 105
Carl Jung, 39
Carl Rogers, 44
Case History, 111
Checking And Testing. See Also'ritual', See Ritual
Cognitive Behavioural Therapies, 33, 44
Degeneration, 33, 34
Depressive Illness, 116
Diagnoses, 55
Dialectical Behaviour Therapy (DBT), 33, 45
Drug Groups, 69, 81
Drug Trials (Process Of), 76 - 80
Eating Disorder, 111, 122
Electro Convulsive Therapy (ECT), 69, 70
Empathy, 59, 62
Encounter Groups, 44
Evidence Based Treatments, 14
Exclusion, 1, 4
Feared Mental Illnesses, 7
Fritz Perls, 44
Frontal Lobes, 37
Hallucination, 82
Hippocrates, 23, 27
Hypnosis, 33, 38
Insanity, 1, 10
Intolerance, 1
Labelling, 1, 6
Largactil, 33, 43
Lazar Houses, 23, 31

Leucotomy, 37
Lithium, 33, 43
Mania, 111, 125
MAOI's (Monoamine Oxidase Inhibitors, 84
Medical Practitioners, 65, 69
Melancholia, 33, 36
Mental Health Act 1983, Xi, 49
Mental Health Rehabilitation Worker, 59, 62
Milton Erickson, 33, 44
Moral Panics, 1, 3
Obsessive Compulsive Disorder (OCD), 111, 129
Persistent Images, 130
Persistent Thoughts, 130
Personality Disorder, 131
Pharmacist, 66
Phobia, 134
Prejudice, 1
Primitive Belief, 23
Psychiatrist, 65
Psychosurgery, 33, 37, 69, 85
Registered Mental Nurse, 66
Samaritans, 107
Schizophrenia, 111, 137
Serotonin And Noradrenaline, 84
Sigmund Freud, 38
Social Work, 64
Stimulant, 82
Stress, 16, **155**
Therapeutic Communities, Xi, 105
Therapist, 59
Thomas Szaz, 45
Trepanning, 23, 24
Tricyclic Antidepressant, 84
Tricyclics, 84
Valium, 33, 43

60268933R00110

Made in the USA
Lexington, KY
01 February 2017